Migraine Headache Prevention and Management

Migraine Headache Prevention and Management

edited by

Seymour Diamond
DIAMOND HEADACHE CLINIC, LTD.
CHICAGO, ILLINOIS

MARCEL DEKKER, INC.   New York and Basel

Library of Congress Cataloging-in-Publication Data

Migraine headache prevention and management / edited by Seymour Diamond.
     p. cm.
  Includes bibliographical references.
  ISBN 0-8247-8212-7 (alk. paper)
  1. Migraine. I. Diamond, Seymour
  [DNLM: 1. Migraine--prevention & control. 2. Migraine--therapy. WL 344 M6357]
RC392.M575 1990
616.8'57--dc20
DNLM/DLC
for Library of Congress   90-3147
                                                                                          CIP

This book is printed on acid-free paper.

Copyright © 1990 MARCEL DEKKER, INC. All Rights Reserved.

Neither this book nor any part may be reproduced or transmitted in any form or by any means, electronic or mechanical, including photocopying, microfilming, and recording, or by any information storage and retrieval system, without permission in writing from the publisher.

MARCEL DEKKER, INC.
270 Madison Avenue, New York, New York 10016

Current printing (last digit):
10 9 8 7 6 5 4 3 2 1

PRINTED IN THE UNITED STATES OF AMERICA

Migraine Headache Prevention and Management

edited by

Seymour Diamond
DIAMOND HEADACHE CLINIC, LTD.
CHICAGO, ILLINOIS

MARCEL DEKKER, INC.   New York and Basel

Library of Congress Cataloging-in-Publication Data

Migraine headache prevention and management / edited by Seymour Diamond.
     p. cm.
  Includes bibliographical references.
  ISBN 0-8247-8212-7 (alk. paper)
  1. Migraine. I. Diamond, Seymour
  [DNLM: 1. Migraine--prevention & control. 2. Migraine--therapy. WL 344 M6357]
RC392.M575 1990
616.8'57--dc20
DNLM/DLC
for Library of Congress   90-3147
                                                                                    CIP

This book is printed on acid-free paper.

Copyright © 1990 MARCEL DEKKER, INC. All Rights Reserved.

Neither this book nor any part may be reproduced or transmitted in any form or by any means, electronic or mechanical, including photocopying, microfilming, and recording, or by any information storage and retrieval system, without permission in writing from the publisher.

MARCEL DEKKER, INC.
270 Madison Avenue, New York, New York 10016

Current printing (last digit):
10 9 8 7 6 5 4 3 2 1

PRINTED IN THE UNITED STATES OF AMERICA

Foreword

*If you would test the skills of a
young physician, give him a patient
with headache to treat.**

It is probable that ever since Homo sapiens learned to communicate, one of the species' most frequent statements has been "I have a headache." It continues to be heard with the persistence of a drumbeat and has been twisted in its significance by the psyche of the speaker. For some it represents an excuse for escape from responsibility. For others it is used as a manipulative tool so that affectionate sympathy can be converted into subservience. But for the sufferer from real migraine, discouraged, agonizing in pain, it is an urgent and prayerful appeal for help.

To this end, scientists through the ages have sought an understanding of the nature of this disorder—the disturbance of body function that produces the disastrous denouement of complete and excruciating disability. The solution of the mystery eludes us, but, sooner or later, all the tiny pieces of the puzzle—identified one at a time by the meticulous labors of a handful of dedicated

---

*William Sunderman, M.D., Professor of Public Health, University of Michigan, 1935.

investigators—will fall together and someone will joyfully shout "Eureka!"

Until that great day, physicians must content themselves—and the patients must be satisfied—with control rather than cure. William Sunderman, M.D. defined disease as "an incompatibility with one's environment." Certainly the migraine sufferer—half blind, nauseated, depressed, in agony—is incompatible with the environment. This includes not only time, place, climate, and light conditions but also the family. In this situation, every therapeutic tool must be marshaled to the effort and used with skill, patience, and forbearance. The available "tools" and their appropriate uses are herein described. It is obvious from their wide variety that no single therapeutic regimen can suffice. The list runs the gamut from the narcotic to the vasoconstrictor and the mind-adjusting. We are now at a stage where control is possible but cure eludes us.

Many of these advances—bringing the problem of headache out of the realm of trephine, mumbo jumbo, and simple analgesics into an area of specific and logical treatment—represent the result of a team effort. Groups of physicians of international scope are meeting at regular intervals to exchange altruistically their ideas and the results of their labors so that each may build upon the work of the others and then "The Cause" can be advanced. A few countries come, at once, to mind: Australia, Canada, Italy, United Kingdom, Scandinavia, Switzerland, and Japan, for example.

This volume represents a distillate of the available "tools." To them must be added the affectionate support, patience, artistry, and dedication of the physician. Without that, they become only "tinkling cymbals."

Perry S. MacNeal, M.D.
Professor of Medicine
University of Pennsylvania
Former President and Distinguished Clinician
American Association for the Study of Headache

Preface

Estimates place the incidence of migraine in the United States at 16 to 18 million sufferers. The economic and personal consequences are abysmal. During the 35 years in which I have been involved in the treatment of migraineurs, a metamorphosis has developed in the "headache world." Initially, the headache conferences that I visited were scarcely attended. Only minor interest was generated in the majority of physicians despite the relevance, frequency, and impact of headache. Books on the subject were limited to a few classics, and journals, for the most part, provided a dearth of coverage on this important topic. This cursory review was partially due to a misconception about the disorder, coupled with a lack of effective therapies.

In the past 10 years, a new understanding of both the mechanisms and effective management has evolved with an awakened interest in the medical community regarding migraine treatment. Thus, we have deemed this period a timely and appropriate opportunity to recruit a group of eminent experts to review the current and practical aspects of both migraine cognition and treatment. It is my hope that this book will stimulate the reader to obtain an enhanced understanding and motivation in adequately treating these patients with newer pharmacological and behavioral modalities.

Seymour Diamond

Contents

Foreword	*iii*
Preface	*v*
Contributors	*xiii*

1. Diagnosis and Pathophysiology of Migraine — 1
Seymour Solomon and Richard B. Lipton

Introduction	1
Diagnosis of Migraine	2
Pathophysiology of Migraine	12
References	25

2. Precipitating Causes of Migraine — 31
R. Michael Gallagher

Introduction	31
Diet	32
Hormonal Influences on Migraine	38
Weather	40
Altitude Changes	41
Psychological Factors	41
Exertion	42
Environmental	43
References	43

3. **Abortive Treatment of Migraine** — 45
   Robert S. Kunkel
   Introduction — 45
   Nonpharmacologic Therapy — 46
   Vasoconstrictive Agents — 46
   Ergotamine-Rebound Headache — 50
   Analgesics — 51
   Sedatives and Antiemetics — 52
   Corticosteroids — 52
   Status Migrainosus — 53
   Aura Without Headache (Migraine Equivalents) — 53
   Summary — 54
   References — 54

4. **The Use of Beta Blockers in Migraine** — 57
   Frederick G. Freitag
   Introduction — 57
   Pharmacology — 57
   Beta Subtype Selectivity — 58
   Partial Agonist Activity — 59
   Serotonin Antagonistic Effect — 59
   Central Nervous System Penetration — 60
   Membrane-Stabilizing Activity — 60
   Cerebral Circulation — 60
   Autonomic Dysregulation — 61
   Central Catecholamine Actions — 62
   Platelet Studies — 63
   Plasma Levels — 64
   Pharmacologic Summary — 65
   Summary — 88
   Conclusions — 90
   References — 91

5. **The Use of Calcium Channel Blockers in Migraine** — 99
   Glen D. Solomon
   Introduction — 99
   The Role of Calcium in Vascular Smooth Muscle — 99
   Pharmacology of Calcium Channel Blockers — 101

Contents

	Comparisons of Calcium Channel Blockers	115
	Conclusion	118
	References	119
6.	**Additional Pharmaceutical Agents Used in Migraine Prophylaxis**	127
	Arthur H. Elkind	
	Introduction	127
	Serotonin Antagonists	128
	Antiplatelet Aggregating Agents	134
	Nonsteroidal Anti-Inflammatory Agents (NSAIDs)	137
	Ergot Alkaloids	141
	Serotonin Precursors	145
	Dopaminergic Agonists	145
	Miscellaneous Agents	146
	Summary	147
	References	149
7.	**Complicated Migraine and Migraine Equivalents**	157
	Donald J. Dalessio	
	Introduction	157
	Migraine with Prolonged Aura (MPA)	158
	(Familial) Hemiplegic Migraine	158
	Basilar Migraine	159
	Ophthalmoplegic Migraine	161
	Retinal Migraine	163
	Migrainous Infarction and Migraine Accompaniments	163
	Treatment of Complicated Migraine	166
	Migraine Equivalents	167
	Treatment of Migraine Equivalents	169
	Summary	169
	References	169
8.	**Management of Migraine in the Elderly**	173
	John Edmeads	
	Introduction	173
	What Kind of Headaches Do the Elderly Have?	174
	Problems of Treating Migraine in the Elderly	183

	Summary	186
	References	187
9.	**Migraine in Childhood**	189
	A. David Rothner	
	Introduction	189
	History	189
	Epidemiology	190
	Classification and Etiology	191
	The Evaluation	191
	Pathophysiology	194
	The Migraine Syndrome	195
	The Migraine Substrate	196
	Types of Migraine	198
	Migraine Variants	202
	Treatment	204
	Prognosis	208
	References	209
10.	**Biofeedback Therapy for Migraine**	213
	Frank Andrasik, Oliver N. Oyama, and Russell C. Packard	
	Introduction	213
	Biofeedback in Relation to Medical Therapy	219
	Mechanisms of Biofeedback Therapy	222
	Considerations in Selecting Patients for Treatment	224
	Considerations in Selecting Biofeedback Therapists	230
	Biofeedback in the Larger Context	232
	Summary	233
	References	234
11.	**Migraine—Unproven Therapeutic Measures**	239
	Richard C. Peatfield	
	Introduction	239
	Feverfew	239
	Air Ionization	243
	Building Sickness	244
	Food Allergy	245

Hypoglycemia	246
Treatment of Neck Structures	247
Temporomandibular Joint Disease	249
Manipulation of Plasma Lipids	249
Acupuncture	250
Marijuana	251
Surgical Treatment	252
References	252

Index *259*

Contributors

Frank Andrasik, Ph.D.[*] Professor and Director of Graduate Studies, Department of Psychology, University of West Florida, Pensacola, Florida

Donald J. Dalessio, M.D. Senior Consultant, Division of Neurology, and Chairman Emeritus, Department of Medicine, Scripps Clinic and Research Foundation, La Jolla, California

John Edmeads, M.D. Professor of Medicine (Neurology), University of Toronto, Toronto, Ontario, Canada

Arthur H. Elkind, M.D. Director, Elkind Headache Center, Mount Vernon, and Clinical Assistant Professor of Medicine, Department of Medicine, New York Medical College, Valhalla, New York

---

Present affiliations:
[*]Professor and Chair, Department of Psychology, Center for Behavioral Medicine, University of West Florida, Pensacola, Florida

Frederick G. Freitag, D.O. Associate Director, Diamond Headache Clinic, Ltd., and Clinical Associate, Department of Internal Medicine, Pritzker School of Medicine, University of Chicago, Chicago, Illinois

R. Michael Gallagher, D.O.[*] Associate Director, Diamond Headache Clinic, Ltd., Chicago, Illinois

Robert S. Kunkel, M.D. Head, Section of Headache, Department of Internal Medicine, Cleveland Clinic Foundation, Cleveland, Ohio

Richard B. Lipton, M.D. Co-Director of Headache Unit, Department of Neurology, Montefiore Medical Center, and Associate Professor of Neurology, Albert Einstein College of Medicine, Bronx, New York

Oliver N. Oyama, Ph.D.[†] Clinical Director, The Avalon Center, Inc., Milton, Florida

Russell C. Packard, M.D., F.A.C.P. Director, Neurology and Headache Management Center, and Adjunct Professor, Department of Psychology, University of West Florida, Pensacola, Florida

Richard C. Peatfield, M.D., M.R.C.P.[‡] Senior Registrar in Neurology, Department of Neurology, St. James University Hospital, Leeds, England

---

Present affiliations:
[*]Director, University Headache Center, School of Osteopathic Medicine, University of Medicine and Dentistry of New Jersey, Stratford, New Jersey
[†]Director, Behavioral Science Education, Duke/FAHEC Family Medicine Residency Program, Fayetteville, North Carolina
[‡]Consultant Neurologist, Department of Neurology, Charing Cross Hospital, London, England

Contributors

A. David Rothner, M.D. Director, Child Neurology, Departments of Neurology and Pediatrics, Cleveland Clinic Foundation, Cleveland, Ohio

Glen D. Solomon, M.D., F.A.C.P. Section of Headache, Department of Internal Medicine, Cleveland Clinic Foundation, Cleveland, Ohio

Seymour Solomon, M.D. Director of Headache Unit, Department of Biology, Montefiore Medical Center, and Professor of Neurology, Albert Einstein College of Medicine, Bronx, New York

1

Diagnosis and Pathophysiology of Migraine

Seymour Solomon and Richard B. Lipton *Montefiore Medical Center and Albert Einstein College of Medicine, Bronx, New York*

INTRODUCTION

Traditionally, pathophysiologic headaches are divided into two groups: those thought to be due to muscle contraction (tension headaches) and those thought to have a vascular mechanism (migraine and cluster headaches). However, there is a growing belief that migraine and tension headaches may be part of the same spectrum. Ostfeld (1) noted that at headache onset, many patients experienced discrete attacks of migraine. With the passage of years, the severity of pain diminished, associated gastrointestinal symptoms waned, and background headaches with characteristics of tension headaches occurred, often daily. A more recent study (2) reaffirmed this sequence. The study found that headache patients with relatively infrequent episodic headaches usually had features of migraine including nausea, those with more frequent headaches had fewer associated features, and those with daily headaches only rarely had features of migraine. This headache-spectrum concept is supported by the clinical overlap between migraine and tension headaches, their response to similar therapy, and research evidence suggesting common mechanisms. Many patients with migraine experience other, less well defined headaches either between attacks of migraine (interval headaches) or mixed with symptoms of migraine (mixed headaches).

In this chapter, we will consider the diagnosis and pathophysiology of migraine. Diagnosis rests on the presence of characteristic clinical features in the headache history. These features are the phenomena that must be explained in considerations of migraine pathogenesis. Because there is no animal model for migraine, much of the data relevant to migraine pathogenesis are derived from the study of human beings with headache disorders. We will consider the human biochemical and physiologic data, as well as the recent animal work on the neurovascular system that has contributed to our understanding of the pathophysiology of migraine.

DIAGNOSIS OF MIGRAINE
History of the Patient

The diagnosis of pathophysiologic headaches is based on a meticulous history of the patient. The examination and laboratory investigations are normal and are undertaken mainly to exclude alternative diagnoses. Evaluation of the important historical features usually will allow the examiner to establish the diagnosis. The age and sex of the patient and the age at headache onset should be considered. The location, quality, and severity of the head pain are important. The duration and frequency of headache, as well as the time of onset, also are helpful. Associated features referable to the central nervous system and the body are extremely important in establishing the diagnosis. Factors that precipitate or aggravate the headache, as well as those that ameliorate it, must be determined. Finally, the presence of a positive family history of headache may help to establish the diagnosis. Of course, all other features of the standard history should be obtained: past history of physical illness, psychological status, and social history.

Diagnosis and Pathophysiology of Migraine

Migraine Without Aura (Common Migraine)

The clinical features of migraine are well described in recent texts (3-10). The typical patient with common migraine is a young woman. Migraine most commonly begins in adolescence and young adulthood. However, while it may begin in childhood or midlife, it rarely starts later. Women are affected about four times more commonly than are men. The typical headache is unilateral, predominantly in the area of the temple, has a throbbing quality, and is of moderate to marked severity. Occasionally, the pain may be bilateral or nonthrobbing. Sometimes, migraineurs experience jabs and jolts of momentary pain scattered over the head. Headaches usually last several hours or all day and sometimes persist into a second or third day. When headaches last longer than 72 hours, the term *status migrainosus* is applied. Migraine most often begins after awakening in the morning, but can occur at any time of the day or night. The frequency of attacks is extremely variable. Some people experience only a few attacks during their lifetime, and others may experience several per week; the average migraineur has one to three headaches per month. Whatever the frequency, migraine is, by definition, a recurrent phenomenon. The diagnosis cannot be applied to a first headache. Especially in patients with new onset headaches that resemble migraine, other diagnoses must be considered. Intracranial vascular anomalies and other cerebral lesions may cause headaches that simulate migraine.

The presence of a prodrome, while not invariable, helps support the diagnosis of migraine. Prodromes may occur several hours or days before an attack. They may be quite subtle, noted by the patient or the family only in retrospect. The patient may inexplicably desire sweets or feel unusually tired. The most common prodromata are changes in mood (irritability, euphoria, a desire to withdraw); fatigue and yawning are common, as are speech impairment and neck stiffness. Symptoms often associated with the headache—photophobia, phonophobia, and vague blurring of vision—often occur long before the attack. Less frequent prodromata include cravings for certain foods, thirst, a sense of generalized weakness, and impairment of thought or concentration.

The presence of associated symptoms during the headache is necessary for the diagnosis of migraine. Nausea, photophobia, and phonophobia are most common. When severe, vomiting and abdominal cramps, as well as tenesmus, may occur. Symptoms of osmophobia, photophobia, and phonophobia demonstrate a heightened sensitivity to sensory stimuli in multiple modalities. There may be swelling about the eyes or of the scalp. Urinary frequency may occur during the attack. Pallor of the face is noted much more commonly than is erythema. There often is tenderness of the involved area of the scalp. Sometimes, veins or arteries are prominent over the temple. There may be associated stiffness of the neck. Mental and personality changes are common and are manifested by difficulty in concentration, fatigue, anxiety, nervousness, and irritability. The patient may be depressed during an attack and elated after its termination. The extremities of migraineurs usually are cold and moist; Raynaud's phenomenon occurs more often in migraineurs than in the general population.

After the headache, the patient enters a resolution phase. Patients often feel washed out, and there may be other postdromal symptoms that last for hours or a day or two. Some patients will feel refreshed or euphoric. Others will experience depression or symptoms similar to those listed as prodromal phenomena.

Migraine with Aura (Classic Migraine)

All of the symptoms described above—the prodrome, the headache phase, and the resolution phase—may occur with classic migraine. Classic migraine is distinguished from common migraine by an aura that follows the prodrome but precedes the headache by an average of 20 to 30 minutes. The aura may consist of any neurologic manifestation, most commonly changes in vision, motor function, or sensation. Occasionally, especially in children, the aura is manifested by altered mentation or consciousness. If the aura is typical and stereotyped, the diagnosis of classic migraine is warranted even if the subsequent headache does not have the other characteristic features. By far the most common aura is a positive scotoma, teichopsia, in the form of an arc of scintillating

Diagnosis and Pathophysiology of Migraine 5

scotoma, a zigzag pattern that grows larger with time. Within the arc may be a negative scotoma; i.e., a blind spot. The scotomata may occur within homonymous fields of vision, but this may not be readily discerned by the patient. Homonymous hemianopsia is common with or without teichopsia. Other visual phenomena may occur as the aura of classic migraine. Objects may appear to change in size or shape or may break into a mosaic pattern. Numbness and tingling over one side of the face and arm are the next most common symptoms of aura; occasionally, the sensory symptoms may involve the entire half of the body. Hemiparesis and, if the dominant hemisphere is involved, dysphasia or aphasia may occur as the aura of classic migraine.

Subtypes of classic migraine are classified by the features of the aura and the duration of the focal neurologic defects. If hemiparesis or hemisensory impairment are major features of the aura of classic migraine, the term *hemiplegic migraine* is applied. In approximately half of these cases, there is a family history of similar hemiplegic headaches. Rarely, migraine is associated with retinal ischemia and blurring or blindness of one eye; if this is the case, the term *retinal migraine* is applied. Amaurosis fugax, associated with carotid-artery disease, may produce an identical visual loss, but usually is associated with risk factors for atherosclerosis. On rare occasions, particularly in children, diplopia occurs in association with the headache. The double vision does not necessarily precede the headache and often persists long after the headache has disappeared. This condition is called *ophthalmoplegic migraine* and is probably caused by compression of oculomotor nerves by an edematous internal carotid artery within the cavernous sinus. In patients with headache and diplopia, aneurysm or other mass lesions must be considered.

When symptoms implicate the brain stem or cerebellum rather than the cerebral hemispheres, the condition is termed *basilar migraine*. This type of migraine most commonly occurs in adolescence. The aura may consist of diplopia or bilateral blindness, tinnitus or hearing impairment, or bilateral paresis or paresthesia; there may be perioral numbness, dysarthria, or dysphagia. Nondescript dizziness, characterized as lightheadedness, is a nonspecific, relatively frequent symptom during common migraine headache, but vertigo or ataxia represents the aura of basilar migraine. Faintness and (rarely) true syncope may occur. The aura may consist of a confusioned state, particularly in children.

When focal symptoms or signs persist beyond the headache phase, the term *complicated migraine* is applied. Rarely, focal symptoms persist for more than a day and may become permanent. Migrainous infarction, although rare, has been documented by imaging techniques in many of these cases; very rarely, angiography reveals spasm or occlusion of intracranial arteries.

Transient cerebral (or, less likely, brain-stem or cerebellar) symptoms may occur without subsequent headache, particularly in men in later life. These are *migraine equivalents*, migraine auras without headache. Transient ischemic attacks due to carotid-artery atherosclerosis or other causes must be ruled out.

The aura of migraine typically is not maximal at onset but evolves. The scintillating scotoma and the visual-field defect grow in size. With the passage of time (20 to 30 minutes), a hemisensory impairment may emerge, sometimes followed by hemiparesis with or without aphasia. In contrast, with transient ischemic attacks of embolic origin, the visual or cerebral symptoms characteristically occur suddenly and are maximal at onset. The visual aura of migraine often is distinguished by the presence of prominent positive phenomena such as scintillations and fortification spectra, while amaurosis fugax due to a transient ischemic attack is characterized primarily by a negative phenomenon, visual loss. Occasionally, the aura of migraine may be maximal at onset and characterized by visual loss alone.

There are certain periodic syndromes of childhood that may be precursors of, or associated with, migraine. Children who manifest bouts of cyclic vomiting sometimes develop migraine in later years. The periodic abdominal pain of children may represent abdominal migraine. Alternating hemiplegia of childhood is thought to have a mechanism akin to migraine. Benign paroxysmal vertigo of childhood has a less certain relationship.

Diagnosis and Pathophysiology of Migraine

Provocative Factors

There are a large number of conditions that precipitate or aggravate migraine. Indeed, virtually any change in the internal milieu or the environment may be a factor. The most common factor is menstruation. Other features implicating female hormones include the increased prevalence of migraine in women and its tendency to begin around the time of menarche, resolve around the time of menopause, and remit during pregnancy, particularly during the last two trimesters. Migraine sometimes is exacerbated by pregnancy, especially in the first trimester, and by oral contraceptives. Abnormal hormonal patterns have not been demonstrated, suggesting that migraineurs have an altered response to hormones rather than abnormalities of hormone production. Some women experience attacks only with menstruation—*menstrual migraine*.

Physical stress such as straining or coughing may aggravate the headache. Relatively minor head trauma or sexual activity may precipitate an attack. Migraine typically occurs during periods of relaxation—after, rather than during, a period of emotional stress. Therefore, an attack may occur after a stressful confrontation with one's employer, on weekends, or during vacations. Missing a meal, too much sleep, or too little sleep are known to be precipitating factors in some instances; these changes may account for the predominance of attacks on weekends in some patients. Head movement or bending over may aggravate the headache. High altitude can bring on migraine. Change in weather is a notable migraine precipitant. And, heat and humidity are more provocative than is cold.

Foods provoke headaches in 8% to 10% of migraineurs. Foods that evoke vasodilation—such as alcoholic beverages, processed meats (containing nitrates), and monosodium glutamate (MSG)—may precipitate attacks. Beer and red wine are more provocative than are other alcoholic beverages, perhaps because of their relatively high tyramine content; the same is true for hard cheeses and herring. The phenylethylamine in chocolate may be a provoking agent. Citrus fruits and nuts commonly initiate migraine. Some data suggest that the sweetener aspartame may trigger migraine, though its role is controversial. Caffeine overuse and caffeine withdrawal also may precipitate headaches.

Medication may provoke migraine, particularly vasodilators (such as nitroglycerine) and reserpine. Contraceptive medication is not absolutely contraindicated in migraineurs, but if the headaches become more prominent during the administration of these agents, they should be discontinued. An important factor that may aggravate migraine and cause its evolution into chronic daily headaches is the abuse of headache medication. Analgesics such as aspirin and acetaminophen, alone or in prescription compounds containing caffeine or barbiturates, are the most common offending agents. Ergotamine compounds, commonly used in the abortive and prophylactic therapy of migraine, also are subject to abuse and may paradoxically lead to daily headaches. The use of sympathomimetic street drugs, including cocaine and amphetamines, also may trigger migraine.

During a migraine attack, patients feel best while lying down in a quiet, dark room. If they can fall asleep, they often awaken refreshed. Compression of the area of the scalp affected by the pain or hot or cold compresses sometimes are helpful. An attack of migraine will disappear spontaneously or in response to medication. Two features often associated with resolution of migraine are sleep and, especially in children, vomiting.

History of Prior Treatment

Other features of the history are important, especially in choosing optimal therapy. A list of all medications taken in the past and details of present medication are essential. Therapeutic effects and side effects should be noted. The pattern of use must be considered, because patients who have received a particular medication may not have had an adequate therapeutic trial. The drug may have been given in suboptimal doses, or the patient may not have taken the drug at the appropriate time. For example, the patient may have used ergots after the headaches were well established,

Diagnosis and Pathophysiology of Migraine

rather than as abortive agents. Details of the past medical history are important, particularly with regard to medications that should be avoided. For example, beta-adrenergic blockers are contraindicated in patients who have asthma and must be used cautiously in diabetic patients. Tricyclic antidepressants are relatively contraindicated in patients who have heart block, a history of mania, or angle-closure glaucoma.

Family, Social, and Psychological History

Finally, the patient's family, social, and psychological history is obtained. The family history of migraine helps support the diagnosis; 75% of migraineurs have a first-degree relative with migraine. Details of marital status, occupation, and social life will permit insight to psychological factors that may precipitate or aggravate headaches. The typical migraine patient often is characterized as a hard-driving, hard-working, well-organized, perfectionistic individual. Patients may be tense and easily upset, yet may not be assertive and may not express their feelings. Depression is associated with many chronic pain syndromes, including migraine. Insomnia, frequent awakening, fatigue on arising in the morning, and other sleep disturbances may be somatic manifestations of underlying depression; these disturbances in themselves may aggravate the attacks. Other manifestations of depression—such as anorexia, constipation, and impaired libido—may be more obvious than are feelings of hopelessness or depressed mood.

Diagnostic Criteria

The most widely used classification and criteria of headache disorders were established in 1962 (11). Recently, a committee of the International Headache Society (IHS) formulated new classification and diagnostic criteria for headache disorders, cranial neuralgias, and facial pain (12). These criteria were established primarily to set a uniform formula for clinical research that would gain worldwide acceptance. The IHS diagnostic criteria for migraine without aura (common migraine) are:

1. At least five attacks fulfilling criteria 2, 3, and 4
2. Headache attacks last 2 to 72 hours
3. Headache has at least two of the following characteristics:
   a. Unilateral location
   b. Pulsating quality
   c. Moderate or severe intensity
   d. Aggravation by routine physical activity
4. During headache, at least one of the following occurs:
   a. Nausea and/or vomiting
   b. Photophobia and phonophobia
5. The history and examinations do not suggest an organic or metabolic disorder, or the latter is ruled out by appropriate investigations, or the migraine attacks do not occur for the first time in close temporal relation to an organic or metabolic disorder.

Though these criteria should be of great value in headache research, they have not been validated empirically. They were designed to be underinclusive rather than overinclusive. While appropriate for research, where it is essential to identify clinically homogeneous patient groups, these criteria may be too restrictive for clinical practice. In practice, the diagnosis helps the clinician to select therapy and advise the patient about prognosis. A less rigorous standard may be appropriate.

Pari passu with the work of the IHS classification committee, we at the Headache Unit of Montefiore Medical Center evaluated 100 consecutive patients diagnosed as having common migraine and compared their symptoms with 100 cases of chronic daily headache (13). We chose chronic daily headache because, based on its frequency, it is the only form of tension headache that unequivocally can be differentiated from migraine. In formulating our criteria, we used those features that occurred significantly more often ($p < .001$) in common migraine than in chronic daily headache. The criteria we proposed for common migraine were:

Recurring idiopathic headache associated with at least two of the following:

1. Nausea with or without vomiting
2. Unilateral pain

Diagnosis and Pathophysiology of Migraine

3. Throbbing quality
4. Photophobia or phonophobia
5. Increase with menses *and* a positive family history of headache

Although they are less rigorous than the IHS criteria, these criteria were derived empirically. We believe that they provide more flexibility than the IHS criteria and should be easier to use in clinical practice. They differ from the IHS criteria in several ways. We did not include the degree of pain as a criterion because gradation of pain is very subjective. While moderate to severe degrees of pain occurred more frequently in patients with migraine than in patients with chronic daily headaches ($p < .01$), the overlap was substantial. Aggravation of headache by routine physical activity was not included because this phenomenon may be related to the severity of pain rather than to the type of headache and has not been studied. We combined headache increased with menstruation and a positive family history of headache into a single criterion to increase specificity. Perhaps these features should be evaluated separately in future studies.

The IHS diagnostic criteria for migraine with aura (classic migraine) are:

1. At least two attacks fulfilling criterion 2
2. At least three of the following four characteristics:
   a. One or more fully reversible aura symptoms indicating cerebral cortical and/or brain-stem dysfunction
   b. At least one aura symptom develops gradually over more than 4 minutes or two or more symptoms occur in succession
   c. No aura symptom lasts more than 60 minutes (if more than one aura symptom is present, accepted duration is proportionally increased)
   d. Headache follows aura with a free interval of less than 60 minutes (it also may begin before or simultaneously with aura)

3. History and examination do not suggest an organic or metablic disorder, or the latter is ruled out by appropriate investigations, or the migraine attacks do not occur for the first time in close temporal relation to an organic or metabolic disorder (12)

Again, these criteria should be very useful in headache research, but require empirical validation.

PATHOPHYSIOLOGY OF MIGRAINE

We do not know the precise mechanisms involved in the cascade of events that produce the migraine syndrome. There are no animal models of migraine. Therefore, our concepts are based primarily on the systemic study of migraineurs using clinical observation, biochemical measurements, and a variety of physiologic techniques. In addition, anatomic and physiologic observations in experimental animals have been used to help understand this exclusively human phenomenon. Though migraine was once viewed as a vascular phenomenon, recent data have suggested a primary role for the nervous system; more particularly, the trigeminovascular system. A comprehensive view of migraine pathogenesis must encompass both neuronal and vascular factors, as well as the neurochemical systems through which they interact.

Classic migraine appears to be initiated by neuronal or biochemical events that lead to the aura and, later, the headache with associated features. Many researchers believe that the headache phase of common migraine and classic migraine share similar mechanisms. In this view, common migraine and classic migraine differ in degree, not kind. In classic migraine, a threshold is crossed and an aura results; in common migraine, the threshold to evoke brain dysfunction is not reached. It also is possible that these conditions are pathophysiologically distinct (14).

Vascular Theories of Migraine

Soon after the discovery of the circulation system by Harvey in the 17th century, a vascular mechanism for migraine was postulated. Willis (15) believed that migraine was due to an excessive amount

Diagnosis and Pathophysiology of Migraine

of blood in the head. Liveing (16) also discussed congestion of the brain, but in addition, proposed a theory of "nerve storms." Latham (17) was the first to suggest a model based on vasoconstriction followed by vasodilation. He proposed "a contraction of the vessels of the brain ... produced by excited action of the sympathetic; and the exhaustion of the sympathetic ... causes dilation of the vessels and the headache." Wolff and his associates (18) elaborated on that basic concept in the 1930s and 1940s. They showed that scalp vessels were dilated during the headache phase. Dilation was associated with increased blood-vessel permeability and exudation of bradykinin and proteolytic enzymes that evoked a perivascular sterile inflammatory reaction, the pain stimulus. In this view, vasospasm causes the aura of migraine, and reactive vasodilation and inflammation initiate the headache. Heyck (19) in the 1950s proposed arteriovenous shunting as the mechanism of the aura and headache. According to this view, the opening of the arteriovenous shunts causes dilation of large veins and arteries, at the expense of capillary flow. The decrease in capillary perfusion would account for the aura of classic migraine, as well as facial pallor, while dural venous dilation would account for the headache (20). Although there may be only a relatively small number of arteriovenous anastamoses in the human brain, they may be hemodynamically significant because the potential ratio of shunt to capillary flow is 10,000 to 1. Nevertheless, there is more evidence against this concept than for it (21).

The early cerebral blood-flow studies tended to support the concept of vasoconstriction and ischemia being responsible for the aura, and vasodilation initiating the events associated with headache (22). However, the decrease in cerebral blood flow usually was not sufficient to cause neuronal ischemia, and subsequent increase in cerebral blood flow did not necessarily correlate with the time of the headache or relate to a similar increase in blood flow of the extracranial circulation, the presumed site of headache.

Platelets and Migraine

Platelet dysfunction has been invoked in the pathophysiology of migraine. Increased platelet adhesiveness and increased platelet aggregation are found in migraineurs between attacks and during the prodrome of migraine (23,24). The sludging of blood elements in low-flow areas of oligemia might be enhanced by platelet hyperaggregability, producing obstruction of microcirculation and neuronal ischemia as a substrate of the aura of classic migraine. Serotonin, thromboxane A, and other vasoactive compounds released by platelets might further impair local cerebral blood flow by causing vasoconstriction or enhancing platelet aggregation. Free fatty acids mobilized by noradrenaline may activate platelets to release serotonin. Bradykinin, histamine, and other polypeptides may act in concert with serotonin, affecting vascular tone and increasing the sensitivity of the blood-vessel wall to nociceptive mechanisms. However, most researchers believe that platelets play a secondary role in migraine pathogenesis (25).

Regulation of Cerebrovascular Tone and Blood Flow

Cerebrovascular tone appears to be regulated by constrictor alpha-adrenergic innervation and dilator beta-adrenergic innervation. Serotonergic, cholinergic, and peptidergic neurons also are important. Within the blood-vessel wall, adenosine, prostaglandin, and other compounds regulate cerebral blood-vessel tone. Other putative neurotransmitters associated with the rich innervation of pial and cerebral blood vessels also have been implicated in the control of cerebral blood flow; for example, substance P, neuropeptide Y, vasoactive intestinal polypeptide (VIP), and calcitonin gene-related peptide (26).

The regulation of cerebrovascular tone depends in part on the local metabolic state through a set of mechanisms referred to as *autoregulation*. When metabolic activity exceeds the oxygen supply, local vasodilation is produced by the accumulation of carbon dioxide and potassium, the development of acidosis, and the decrease in oxygen tension. The consequent increase in blood flow tends to restore metabolic balance.

Neural Theories of Migraine

For more than a century, the aura of migraine was thought to be a consequence of cerebral ischemia, caused by vascular changes as

Diagnosis and Pathophysiology of Migraine

the primary event. Emerging evidence suggests that neural events may be primary and changes in blood flow secondary. The changes in mood, appetite, and other phenomena noted for hours or days before an attack (and similar symptoms that may follow the headache) are best explained by altered brain function. These events favor a neural rather than a vascular mechanism.

The Aura and Spreading Depression

Modern neural concepts of migraine began in 1944 with Leao's discovery of spreading depression of cortical neuronal activity (27, 28). A localized stimulus to the rabbit cerebral cortex evokes a wave of depolarization that causes depression of neuronal activity spreading in all directions, without regard to arterial territory or neuronal pathways. Lashley (29) plotted the duration and path of the scintillating scotomas he experienced during his own migraine auras and calculated that the changes must spread over the occipital cortex at an approximate rate of 3 mm/min. Later, it was noted that spreading depression moves over the cortical surface at a similar rate (30). Moreover, the cortical neurons on the leading margin of spreading depression were markedly activated (31). This neuronal discharge could account for photopsia, the positive scintillations, while the spreading neuronal depression could account for the negative scotoma or homonymous hemianopsia of the migraine aura. The typical aura evolves over time and space. It may spread from the occipital to the parietal and then to the frontal cortex, but it notably does not conform to the distribution of a single major arterial territory. A carbon dioxide-oxygen mixture stops spreading depression in the rat cortex (32); it sometimes stops the aura or headache in people.

More recently, Lauritzen et al. (14,33) performed serial cerebral blood-flow studies during the aura of classic migraine and showed that a decrease in blood flow progressed from the posterior to anterior direction over the cerebral cortex at a rate of change roughly corresponding to that of the spreading depression reported by Leao. Other correlations of cerebral blood-flow changes with the spreading depression of neuronal activity have been emphasized (34). According to this view, the decrease in cerebral blood flow is a consequence of decreased metabolic demand due to depression of neuronal activity. In other words, the decrease in blood flow reflects primary changes in neuronal function, not vasoconstriction and ischemia.

Positron emission tomography (PET) also has yielded interesting data with regard to the sequence and duration of oligemia and hyperemia during migraine. Oligemia extends into, and hyperemia often extends beyond, the headache phase of the attack (35). PET eventually may differentiate between the two proposed mechanisms of the aura of migraine. If the brain dysfunction is due to vasoconstriction causing ischemia, the PET studies should reveal an increase in the oxygen-extraction fraction (as the brain attempts to maintain maximum viability). If the brain dysfunction is due to spreading depression of neuronal activity with diminished regional cerebral blood flow secondary to decreased metabolic demands, the oxygen-extraction fraction should be normal or perhaps slightly diminished.

There is one major problem with the concept of spreading depression as the mechanism of migraine. Spreading depression is evoked easily in the cortex of lower animals, but is difficult to evoke in monkeys and, with one possible exception (36), has not been demonstrated in humans. Corticography during epilepsy surgery has provided ample opportunity to demonstrate spreading depression, but it has not been observed. Perhaps the brains and cranial blood vessels of migraineurs differ from those of the rest of the population in their susceptibility to spreading depression. Alternatively, the prelude to classic migraine may create circumstances that are uniquely able to evoke spreading depression.

The Headache and the Trigeminal Nerve

The pain of migraine may be influenced by several factors. It had been assumed that the nociceptive impulses from blood vessels of the head were carried by the trigeminal nerve. Recent data support this concept. In the cat, electrical stimulation of the face and of dural arteries evokes responses recorded from the trigeminal brain-stem nucleus (subnucleus caudalis) (37). Labeled horseradish peroxidase (HRP), when applied to the middle cerebral artery of

Diagnosis and Pathophysiology of Migraine 17

the cat, undergoes retrograde axonal transport to cell bodies in the medial portion of the ipsilateral trigeminal ganglion (corresponding to the first division of the trigeminal in man) (38). Similar findings were noted when HRP was applied to the dural arteries and sinuses.

The first division of the trigeminal nerve innervates all the major cerebral arteries, including the upper basilar artery, and the extracranial blood vessels. The perivascular fibers of the trigeminal nerve also serve as an interface between the circulation and the brain. Trigeminal nerve stimulation (in the cat) results in carotid dilation and an increase in regional cerebral blood flow through connections made with the facial nerve nucleus and its pathways (39). Thus, in migraineurs, the trigeminal nerve provides the afferent system for head pain and a mechanism for linking neuronal and vascular changes; its stimulation may evoke carotid dilation, probably via autonomic impulses through the nervus intermedius (40). The auriculotemporal syndrome is an example of these phenomena; the efferent neurons in the auriculotemporal branch of the trigeminal nerve are part of the reflex that increases extracranial blood flow.

The Sequence of Aura and Headache

By integrating our knowledge of the trigeminovascular system with the concept of spreading depression, the aura and the headache of migraine may be explained. As the wave of spreading depression propagates over the surface of the brain, it may influence the pain-sensitive arteries innervated by the trigeminal nerve. High extracellular potassium, which develops as a consequence of spreading depression (35), may depolarize trigeminal nerve terminals around pial arteries, releasing substance P and probably other nociceptive neurotransmitters. Substance P may cause the marked dilation of pial arteries and veins in the wake of spreading depression. In addition, this transmitter may increase the permeability of blood vessels, degranulate mast cells, and stimulate prostaglandin synthesis, leading to periarterial inflammation and pain (41). This hypothesis links the aura and the pain of migraine. The aura is caused by neuronal depression, and the headache is caused by the release of substance P from trigeminal terminals of pial arteries.

The Triggering Pathways

A neuronal stimulus most likely precipitates the migraine cascade. Some researchers believe that there is an initial activation of the central sympathetic nervous system that lowers the threshold for migraine activation (42), while others suggest that hypoactivity of the sympathetic nervous system may result in denervation hypersensitivity (43). The peripheral autonomic nervous system is not essential to migraine; sectioning of the cervical sympathetic ganglion or the greater superficial petrosal nerve does not alter this condition (44,45). More important are adrenergic and serotinergic neurons that project from the brain stem to the microcirculation of the cerebral cortex.

The locus ceruleus (a group of neurons ventral to the mesencephalic nucleus and tract of the trigeminal nerve in the midbrain and upper pons) is thought to be the central analogue of the peripheral sympathetic ganglia. Noradrenergic neurons from the locus ceruleus and other brain-stem nuclei project to the cortical microcirculation; low-frequency stimuli of this structure (in the monkey) induce vasoconstriction that often is asymmetrical (46). There is an associated decrease in neural activity, as well as an increase in vascular permeability. Serotonergic neurons whose cell bodies are situated in the midbrain raphe (midline) nucleii (especially nucleus raphe dorsalis) have a similar distribtuion and probably a similar action (47,48). High-frequency stimulation of the locus ceruleus evokes carotid-artery vasodilation via autonomic pathways of the facial nerve (46). (Cholinergic neurons from the pons pass through the nervus intermedius of the facial nerve to the internal carotid artery and its branches and mediate vasodilation, but the effects of locus ceruleus stimulation are not cholinergic.) Note the potential circuit: stimuli from the brain causing constriction of the cortical and dilation of the carotid vessels, triggering nociceptive impulses carried by the trigeminal nerve. Trigeminal nerve stimuli evoke carotid dilation and may increase cerebral blood flow.

Diagnosis and Pathophysiology of Migraine 19

Serotonergic neurons from the nucleus raphe magnus of the brain stem descend and act as inhibitory nociceptive modulators at the enkephalinergic "gate" of primary sensory neurons entering the spinal cord and brain stem. Noradrenergic neurons from the locus ceruleus accompany the descending serotonergic neurons, and their effect on nociception is similar (49). Activation of these centers not only may initiate the aura, but also may initially dampen nociception. Subsequently, as the aura fades, there may be a decrease in the inhibition of nociception, opening the pain gate and perhaps the gate that modulates response to special senses. Sensitivity to light and sound (photophobia and phonophobia), as well as to pain, then may be enhanced

Biochemical Concepts of Migraine

Whether vascular or neuronal mechanisms are primary, we know that neurotransmitters, hormones, and other biochemicals are the ultimate mediators of neural transmission and vascular reactivity. Serotonin and noradrenaline are implicated most often in the pathophysiology of migraine.

Catecholamines and Serotonin

During migraine attacks, Sicuteri (50) found an increase in urinary 5-hydroxyindoleacetic acid (5-HIAA), the major metabolite of serotonin. A drop in blood serotonin during attacks was found to be the most consistent (although not invariable) biochemical change of migraine (51). The action of serotonin varies with the species of the animal and the size of the blood vessel (52). In humans, serotonin causes vasoconstriction of large blood vessels in the external carotid arterial tree, but dilation of small blood vessels; it also induces platelet aggregation and may cause the opening of arteriovenous shunts. It was thought that a decrease in blood serotonin reduces its constrictor effect and leads to vasodilation and headache. The vasoconstrictor effect of serotonin, however, is noted only after large, nonphysiological intravenous dosage (in monkeys) (53). Moreover, serotonin blood levels have little relationship to intracellular serotonin; the observed changes in the blood probably are an epiphenomenon. Almost all the serotonin found in blood is located in the platelets, and platelet release and reabsorption of serotonin may be a model for pre- and post-synaptic functions of serotonergic neurons (54).

The studies of catecholamine metabolism in migraine have not revealed consistent findings (55). Some studies (56) found increased urinary vanillylmandelic acid (VMA), the metabolite of adrenaline and noradrenaline, during headache when compared to the preheadache period, but others (57) failed to confirm this observation. Migraineurs are thought to have increased sympathetic activity (58), even when headache-free. Plasma noradrenaline and adrenaline in headache-free migraineurs are elevated in comparison to a population without migraine (59). However, a rise in plasma noradrenaline in association with migraine attacks simply may be a response to physiological stress. As with serotonin, the serum catecholamine levels may have little to do with the parenchymal actions of these agents.

Substance P

Several polypeptides are found in primary sensory neurons, and activation of these neurons releases nociceptor transmitters that activate or modulate polymodal pain receptors. These compounds also may initiate and perpetuate tissue inflammation, which, in turn, evokes pain. Inflammation, completing a cycle, generates additional polypeptides. Of the polypeptides, substance P has been studied most extensively.

An important biochemical relationship to migraine was reported by Moskowitz et al (60). Substance P is synthesized in nerve cells, and 75% of it is found in afferent processes of the neurons associated with polymodal nociceptive pain transmission. Substance P, measured by radioimmune assay, is found in the trigeminovascular fibers of large arteries in the pia and arachnoid. In addition to its action as a putative neurotransmitter of nociceptive stimuli, release of substance P from perivascular nerve fibers mediates vasodilation, increases vascular permeability, and initiates inflammation (41). This action is thought to be analogous to the

Diagnosis and Pathophysiology of Migraine 21

axon reflex. The relaxation of blood-vessel musculature by substance P is endothelial-dependent, suggesting that dilation is regulated by humoral agents. Other peptides (bradykin, metabolites of arachodonic acid, acetylcholine, and calcium ionophore) also cause vasodilation.

Depolarization of primary sensory trigeminal neurons innervating the eye, skin, and mucosa causes increased permeability of their blood-vessel walls and probably of cerebral blood vessels as well. These reactions are blocked by capsaicin and other antagonists of substance P (41). Hyperpermeability permits exudation of plasma proteins. Earlier studies found that polypeptides in fluid aspirated from tender areas of the scalp during migraine headache had pain-producing qualities; they were termed neurokinin (61). These polypeptides had features similar to substance P and bradykinin.

Substance P affects cells that take part in the inflammatory response: mast cells, polymorphonuclear leukocytes, tissue macrophages, and human T lymphocytes (41). Substance P degranulates mast cells and probably is associated with their release of histamine; it stimulates phagocytosis by polymorphonuclear leukocytes and macrophages, stimulates prostaglandin synthesis in tissue macrophages, and increases tritiated thymidine incorporation into T lymphocytes. (Large doses of substance P also stimulate chemotaxis and lysosomal enzyme secretion.)

Other Biochemicals

Other biochemicals have been implicated in regulation of vascular tone and in the pathogenesis of migraine. These include dopamine, histamine, monoamine oxidase (MAO), adenine compounds, VIPs, prostaglandins, neuropeptide Y, and calcitonin gene-related peptide. If tyramine and phenylethylamine have a role in the pathophysiology of migraine, it is probably as precipitating agents in those patients who relate their attacks to foods containing these agents. While the most consistent change during an attack of migraine is the fall in plasma (platelet) serotonin concentration, there is a rise in plasma levels of some of the other biogenic amines; for example, dopamine and histamine. These compounds also tend to cause vasodilation (not fully countered by a raised level of noradrenaline) (55). While individual effects are weak, the summation of these changes may evoke cranial vasodilation. Polypeptides often work together. Serotonin coexists with substance P in trigeminal ganglia, and the two agents may work in concert. Perhaps serotonin released by platelets, as well as serotonin in nerve fibers around cerebral blood vessels, joins with other biochemicals of the altered blood-vessel wall.

Relevance to Therapy

Agents used for prophylactic migraine therapy interact with the neurochemical systems implicated in migraine pathogenesis. Antiserotonergic agents and beta blockers probably work on central neurons. Prostaglandin inhibitors act on the pain mechanism at the periarterial site and also may modulate noradrenergic function. Calcium-channel blockers interfere with the synaptic calcium-dependent potassium channels, as well as with the passage of calcium ions into smooth muscle cells, thus modulating their contraction. If combination prophylactic therapy is required, it would be sensible to combine agents that act at different sites with the hope of achieving synergistic therapeutic benefits.

The Initiation of a Migraine Attack

What causes migraine? The high familial incidence of migraine indicates genetic susceptibility, but the basic answer to the question is unknown. A good deal, however, is known about factors that trigger an attack.

Changes in the milieu of the central nervous system (CNS) may precipitate migraine, probably by influencing adrenergic and serotonergic neurons. The hormonal changes associated with menstruation may trigger attacks by acting on hormone receptors within the CNS. Alterations in sleep pattern and other factors related to biological clocks also may trigger attacks by altering the milieu of the CNS. Biological clocks regulating menstruation, sleep, and appetite depend, at least in part, on hypothalamic

Diagnosis and Pathophysiology of Migraine

mechanisms. Neurons of the hypothalamus project to the brain stem and, through the limbic system, to the neocortex. Through these systems, the hypothalamus interacts with the autonomic nervous system and modulates sensation, emotional stimuli, and other external factors.

Many external stimuli may trigger a migraine attack. Light, sound, trauma (stretching of blood vessels), sexual activity, change in weather, and emotional stress cause neuronal stimulation. Drugs and foods known to precipitate migraine result in metabolic stimuli. Neuronal stimuli are relayed from the primary cerebral cortex to the orbitofrontal cortex, and from there to centers modulating sensory input, emotional phenomena, and the autonomic nervous system via the thalamus, the temporal lobe and limbic system, and the brain-stem nuclei, respectively.

Whether the precipitant of migraine is an intrinsic metabolite or an extrinsic neural stimulus, it is probably modulated by several factors. For example, metabolic factors such as estrogens, tyramine, and tyrosine (the parent amino acids for norepinephrine synthesis) probably influence the intrinsic adrenergic nervous system. Internal circuits, whether initiated by metabolic or neuronal stimuli, respond (feedback) to changes associated with menstruation, sleep, appetite, and other biological alterations. The stimuli reach brain-stem centers and initiate the cascade of events discussed (neural theories). Feedback occurs via noradrenergic neurons from the locus ceruleus and other brain-stem nuclei, which project to the limbic system and neocortex, influencing the higher processing of sensory perception and cognitive function. Responses to stress are regulated by these circuits.

The Mechanisms of Other Features of Migraine

The unilaterality of migraine is a mysterious phenomenon. One theoretical explanation is a deficiency in migraineurs in the regulation of regional CNS activation, the mechanism for which is probably in the diffuse thalamic projection system (62). Another explanation for the unilaterality of migraine has to do with a theoretical alteration in the number and affinities of trigeminal receptors modified by neuronal or biochemical factors. Systemic administration of estrogen increases the size of the receptive field of trigeminal mechanoreceptors. Perhaps other substances known to precipitate migraine alter the receptive field properties or threshold of trigeminal neurons (41).

Many researchers believe that tension headache and migraine have similar mechanisms. Headaches that fit the criteria of tension headaches commonly occur with or between attacks of migraine. Of the experimental evidence that supports this concept, recent studies (63,64) have found substance P and other putative nociceptive neurotransmitters in human temporal arteries and other scalp tissue. Furthermore, depletion of cerebrospinal fluid (CSF) endorphin (65), decrease in serum serotonin (66), and alteration of other platelet biochemicals (67) have been noted with tension headaches as well as with migraine.

Summary of Neurovascular Biochemical Concepts

Migraine begins when some external or internal change activates primary cortical CNS neurons or the hypothalamus. Impulses then are relayed to the brain stem. The brain-stem noradrenergic and serotonergic neurons evoke cortical microcirculation vasoconstriction, which induces the aura of migraine either by primary ischemia or, more likely, by initiating spreading depression of cortical neuronal activity. At the same time, descending serotinergic and noradrenergic impulses inhibit pain during the aura.

The aura fades after 20 to 30 minutes, and a counterreaction occurs. The wave of spreading depression has reached the trigeminally innervated blood vessels. There is release of substance P, initiating pain transmission and enhancing vasodilation and periarterial inflammation. At about the same time, discharges from the locus ceruleus cause ipsilateral dilation of the extracranial blood vessels via the autonomic pathways in the seventh nerve. There also is a decrease in downward serotonin and norepineprhine transmission, which opens the pain gate.

REFERENCES

1. Ostfeld, A. (1963). The natural history and epidemiology of migraine and muscle contraction headache, *Neurology, 13*: 11-15.
2. Drummond P. D. and Lance, J. W. (1984). Clinical diagnoses and computer analyses of headache symptoms, *J. Neurol. Neurosurg. Psychiatry, 47*:128-133.
3. Barlow, C. F. (1984). *Headaches and Migraine in Childhood*, Blackwell Scientific Publications, Oxford; J. B. Lippincott, Philadelphia.
4. Blau, J. N. (1987). Adult migraine: The patient observed, *Migraine. Clinical and Research Aspects* (J. N. Blau, ed.), The Johns Hopkins University Press, Baltimore, pp. 3-30.
5. Dalessio, D. J. (1987). *Wolff's Headache and Other Head Pain* (5th ed.), Oxford University Press, New York.
6. Diamond, S. and Dalessio, D. J. (1988). *The Practicing Physician's Approach to Headache* (4th ed.), Williams & Wilkins, Baltimore.
7. Lance, J. W. (1982). *Mechanism and Management of Headache* (4th ed.), Butterworth Scientific, Boston.
8. Raskin, N. H. (1988). *Headache* (2nd ed.), Churchill Livingstone, New York.
9. Saper, J. R. (1983). *Headache Disorders. Current Concepts and Treatment Strategies*, John Wright PSG, Boston.
10. Wilkinson, M. (1986). Clinical features of migraine, *Headache*, Vol. 48 of *Handbook of Clinical Neurology* (P. J. Vinken, G. W. Bruyn, H. L. Klawans, and F. C. Rose, eds.) Elsevier Science Publishing, New York, pp. 117-133.
11. Committee on Classification of Headache of the National Institute of Neurological Diseases and Blindness (1962). Classification of Headache, *JAMA, 179*: 717-718.
12. Headache Classification Committee of the International Headache Society (1988). Classification and diagnostic criteria for headache disorders, cranial neuralgias, and facial pain. *Cephalalgia, 8 (Suppl. 7)*: 1-96.
13. Solomon, S., Guglielmo-Cappa, K., and Smith C. R. (1988). Common migraine: Criteria for diagnosis, *Headache, 28*: 124-129.

14. Lauritzen, M., and Olesen, J. (1984). Regional cerebral blood flow during migraine attacks by Xenon-133 inhalation and emission tomography, *Brain, 107*: 447-461.
15. Willis, T. (1686). *Practice of Physick*, London.
16. Liveing, E. (1873). *Megrim. Sick Headache and Some Allied Disorders*, Churchill, London.
17. Latham, P. (1872). Clinical lectures on nervous or sick headaches, *Br. Med. J., 1*: 305-306, 336-337.
18. Wolff, H. G. (1948). *Headache and Other Head Pain*, Oxford University Press, New York.
19. Heyck, H. (1981). *Headache and Facial Pain*, Georg, Thieme Verbag Stuttgart.
20. Rowbotham, G. F. and Little, E. (1965). New concepts in the etiology and vascularization of meningiomata; the mechanism of migraine; the chemical processes of cerebrospinal fluid; and the formation of collections of blood or fluid in the subdural space, *Br. J. Surg., 52*:21-24.
21. Spierings, E. L. H. (1984). The role of arteriovenous shunting in migraine, *The Pharmacological Basis of Migraine Therapy* (W. K. Amery, J. M. Van Nueten, and A. Wanquier, eds.), Pitman, London, pp. 36-49.
22. O'Brien (1971). Cerebral blood changes in migraine, *Headache, 11*: 139-143.
23. Deshmukh, S. V. and Meyer, J. S. (1977). Cyclic changes in platelet dynamics and the pathogenesis and prophylaxis of migraine, *Headache, 17*:101-108.
24. Hannington, E., Jones, R. J., Amess, J. A. L., and Wachowicz, B. (1981). Migraine—a platelet disorder, *Lancet, 2*: 720-723.
25. Steiner, T. J., Joseph, R., and Rose, F. C. (1985). Migraine is not a platelet disorder, *Headache, 25*: 434-440.
26. Lou, H. C., Edvinsson, L. and MacKenzie, E. T. (1987). The concept of coupling blood flow to brain function: Revision required? *Ann. Neurol, 22*: 289-297.
27. Leao, A. A. P. (1944). Spreading depression of activity in the cerebral cortex, *J. Neurophysiol, 7*: 359-390.
28. Leao, A. A. P. (1947). Further observations on the spreading depression of activity in the cerebral cortex, *J. Neurophysiol, 10*: 409-419.
29. Lashley, K. S. (1941). Patterns of cerebral integration indicated by the scotomas of migraine, *Arch. Neurol. Psychiatry, 46*:331-339.

30. Milner, P. M. (1958). Note on a possible correspondence between scotomas of migraine and spreading depression of Leao, *Electroencephalog. Clin. Neurophysiol, 10*: 705.
31. Grafstein, B. (1956). Mechanisms of spreading cortical depression. *J. Neurophysiol., 19*: 308-316.
32. Gardner-Medwin, A. R. (1981). Possible roles of vertebrate neuralgia in potassium dynamics, spreading depression, and migraine, *J. Exp. Biol., 95*: 111-127.
33. Lauritzen, M., Skyhj, T., Lassen, N. A., and Paulson, O. B. (1983). Changes in regional cerebral blood flow during the course of classic migraine attacks, *Ann. Neurol., 13*: 633-641.
34. Lauritzen, M. (1984). Spreading cortical depression in migraine, *The Pharmacological Basis of Migraine Therapy* (W. K. Amery, J. M. Van Neuten, and A. Wanquier, eds.), Pitman, London, pp. 149-160.
35. Andersen, A. R., Friberg, L., Olsen, T. S., and Olesen, J. (1988). Delayed hyperemia following hypoperfusion in classic migraine. Single photon emission computed tomographic demonstration, *Arch. Neurol., 45*: 154-159.
36. Sramka, M., Brozek, G., Bures, J., and Nadvornik, P. (1977-1978). Functional ablation of spreading depression: Possible use in human stereotatic neurosurgery. *Appl. Neurophysiol, 40*: 48-61.
37. Davis, K. D. and Dostrovsky, J. O. (1986). Activation of trigeminal brain stem nociceptive neurons by dural artery stimulation, *Pain, 25*: 395-401.
38. Mayberg, M. R., Zervas, N. T., and Moskowitz, M. A. (1984). Trigeminal projections to supratentorial pial and dural blood vessels in cats demonstrated by horseradish peroxidase histochemistry, *J. Comp. Neurol, 223*: 46-56.
39. Goadsby. P. J. and Duckworth, J. W. (1987). Effect of stimulation of trigeminal ganglion on regional cerebral blood flow in cats, *Am. J. Physiol., 253*: R270-R274.
40. Lance, J. W., Lambert, G. A., Goadsby, P. J., and Duckworth, J. W. (1983). Brain-stem influences on the cephalic circulation: Experimental data from cat and monkey of relevance to the mechanism of migraine, *Headache, 23*: 258-265.
41. Moskowitz, M. A. (1984). The neurobiology of vascular head pain, *Ann. Neurol., 16*: 157-168.

42. Welch, K. M. A., Darnley, D., and Simkins, R. T. (1984). The role of estrogens in migraine: A review and hypothesis, *Cephalalgia, 4*: 227-236.
43. Gotoh, F., Komatsumoto, S., Araki, N., and Gomi, S. (1984). Noradrenergic nervous activity in migraine, *Arch. Neurol., 41*: 951-955.
44. White, J. C. and Smithwick, R. H. (1935). *The Autonomic Nervous System; Anatomy, Physiology and Surgical Treatment.* Macmillan, New York, pp. 255-257.
45. Gardner, W. J., Stowell, A., and Dutlinger, R. (1947). Resection of the greater superficial petrosal nerve in the treatment of unilateral headache, *J. Neurosurg, 4*: 105-114.
46. Goadsby, P. J., Lambert, G. A., and Lance, J. W. (1982). Differential effects on internal and external carotid circulation of the monkey evoked by locus coeruleus stimulation, *Brain Res., 249*: 247-254.
47. Reinhard, J. F., Jr., Liebmann, J. E., Schlosberg, A. J., and Moskowitz, M. A. (1979). Serotonin neurons project to small blood vessels in the brain, *Science, 206*: 85-87.
48. Scatton, B., Duverger, D., L'Heureux, R., et al. (1985). Neurochemical studies on the existence, origin, and characteristics of the serotonergic innervation of small pial vessels, *Brain Res., 345*: 219-229.
49. Fields, H. L. (1987). *Pain*, McGraw-Hill, New York, pp. 99-131.
50. Sicuteri, F., Testi, A., and Anselmi, B. (1961). Biochemical investigations in headache: Increase in hydro-oxyindoleacetic acid excretion during migraine attacks, *Int. Arch. Allergy Appl. Immunol., 19*: 55-58.
51. Anthony, M., Hinterberger, H., and Lance, J. W. (1967). Plasma serotonin in migraine and stress, *Arch. Neurol., 16*: 544-552.
52. MacKenzie, E. T., Edvinsson, L., and Scatton, B. (1985). Functional bases for a central serotonergic involvement in classic migraine: A speculative view, *Cephalalgia, 5*: 69-78.
53. Spira, P. J., Mylecharane, E. J., and Lance, J. W. (1976). The effects of humoral agents and antimigraine drugs on the cranial circulation of the monkey, *Res. Clin. Stud. Headache, 4*:37-75.
54. Mamgren, R. and Hasselmark, L. (1988). The platelet and the neuron: Two cells in focus in migraine, *Cephalalgia, 8*: 7-24.

55. Anthony, M. (1987). Amine metabolism in migraine, *Migraine. Clinical and Research Aspects*, (J. N. Blau, ed.), The Johns Hopkins University Press, Baltimore, pp. 303-329.
56. Sicuteri, F. (1967). Vasoneuroactive substances and their implication in vascular pain, *Res. Clin. Stud. Headache 1*, (A. P. Friedman, ed.), Karger, New York, pp. 6-45.
57. Curzon, C. (1967). Amine changes in migraine, *Background to Migraine* (R. Smith, ed.), Heinemann, London, pp. 134-143.
58. Welch, K. M. A. (1987). Migraine. A behavioral disorder, *Arch. Neurol., 44*: 323-327.
59. Mathew, R. J., Ho, B. T., Kralik, P., Taylor, D., and Glaghorn, J. L. (1980). Catecholamines and migraine: Evidence based on biofeedback induced changes, *Headache, 20*: 247-252.
60. Moskowitz, M. A., Reinhard, J. F., Jr., Romero, J., Melamed, E., and Pettibone, D. J. (1979). Neurotransmitters and the fifth cranial nerve: Is there a relation to the headache phase of migraine? *Lancet, 2*: 883-884.
61. Chapman, L. F., Ramos, A. O., Goodell, H., Silverman, G., and Wolff, H. G. (1960). A humoral agent implicated in vascular headaches of the migraine type, *Arch. Neurol., 15*: 223-229.
62. Gruzelier, J. H., Nicolaou, T., Connolly, J. F., Peatfield, R. C., Davies, P. T. G., and Clifford-Rose, F. (1987). Laterality of pain in migraine distinguished by interictal rates of habituation of electrodermal responses to visual and auditory stimuli, *J. Neurol. Neurosurg. Psychiatry, 50*: 416-422.
63. Jansen, I., Uddman, R., Hocherman, M., et al. (1986). Localization and effects of neuropeptide Y, vasoactive intestinal polypeptide, substance P and calcitonin gene-related peptide in human temporal arteries, *Ann. Neurol., 20*: 496-501.
64. Uddman, R., Edvinsson, L., Jansen, I., et al. (1986). Peptide-containing nerve fibers in human extracranial tissue: A morphological basis for neuropeptide involvement in extracranial pain? *Pain, 27*: 391-399.
65. Genazzani, A. R., Nappi, G., Facchinetti, F., et al. (1984). Progressive impairment of CSF beta-EP levels in migraine sufferers. *Pain, 18*: 127-133.

66. Rolf, L. H., Wiele, G., and Brune, G. G. (1981). 5-Hydroxytriptamine in platelets of patients with muscle contraction headache, *Headache, 21*: 10-11.
67. Takeshima, T., Shimomura, T., and Takahashi, K. (1987). Platelet activation in muscle contraction headache and migraine, *Cephalalgia, 7*: 239-243.

2

Precipitating Causes of Migraine

R. Michael Gallagher* *Diamond Headache Clinic, Ltd., Chicago, Illinois*

INTRODUCTION

Most headache specialists agree that certain factors or conditions tend to precipitate or at least contribute to the frequency and/or severity of migraine headache attacks. Migraine sufferers seem to have an exaggerated reactivity to external and internal stimuli. Some of the more commonly implicated precipitants are diet, hunger, tension, hormonal fluctuation, and irregular sleep. The elimination of the precipitants usually will not prevent headaches completely, but may cause an overall reduction in attack frequency and severity.

**Present affiliation*: School of Osteopathic Medicine, University of Medicine and Dentistry of New Jersey, Stratford, New Jersey

DIET

The relationship between diet and migraine headache has been discussed and argued by physicians and researchers for many years. Although well-controlled, double-blind studies are few, numerous studies and surveys have been conducted by authorities and well-known specialists. Diamond and Blau (1) conducted a survey of 327 physicians who were interested in the headache problem and found that most agreed that migraines can be induces by the intake of certain foods. Although many physicians and patients feel that a relationship does exist, an understanding of this relationship is most difficult and coomplex, since triggering foods vary from patient to patient.

Complicating the diet-migraine matter further is that particular dietary triggers do not always provoke attacks each time they are eaten in given individuals. Migraine attacks can result from a multitude of causative factors, of which diet is only one. Environmental changes, stress, fatigue, and hormonal changes also may play a significant role. Some women report being susceptible to diet-induced migraine only during menses. Other patients report being susceptible only while fatigued or when exposed to strong sunlight.

Some of the foods commonly implicated in diet-related migraine are chocolate, cheese, beans, seafood, nuts, citrus fruits, and onions (see Table 1). These foods contain vasoactive amines such as tyramine, phenylethylamine, dopamine, or histamine. The vasoactive amines are physiologically potent and can affect the body vasculature markedly. In susceptible individuals, small amounts can produce headache. Tyramine is found in a significant number of provocative foods.

Certain food additives such as MSG, sodium nitrite, caffeine, and alcohol also are implicated in provoking migraine. The exact mechanism is not completely understood, but is thought to involve a vasoconstriction-dilation mechanism.

Tyramine

Tyramine is an amino acid with sympathomimetic properties. It is found in many migraine-provoking foodstuffs and is thought to be

TABLE 1 Migraine-Precipitating Foods*

Beverages	Dairy
alcoholic	aged and processed cheese
caffeine (limit to 2 cups/day)	yogurt (limit to ½ cup/day)
chocolate milk	Baked goods
buttermilk	fresh baked breads
Meat/fish	sourdough
pickled herring	Vegetables
chicken livers	fava beans
sausage	lima beans
salami	navy beans
pepperoni	pea pods
bologna	sauerkraut
frankfurters	onions
marinated meats	Desserts
aged, canned, or cured meats	chocolate
Fruits	Other
canned figs	soy sauce
raisins	MSG
papaya	meat tenderizer
passion fruit	seasoning salt
avocado	canned soups
bananas	TV dinners
red plums	garlic
citrus fruits (limit to ½ cup/day)	yeast extracts

*Extracted from the National Headache Foundation Headache Diet, Chicago, Illinois.

nontoxic under usual circumstances. It acts directly on blood vessels and causes the release of endogenous aromatic amines from sympathetic nerve endings and serotonin from platelets (2). This can result in selective cerebral vasoconstriction and subsequent rebound vasodilation (3), causing a headache in susceptible individuals. Tyramine is rapidly metabolized by the liver in normal individuals. However, there is evidence to suggest that migraine patients have an altered ability to degrade it to an inactive form (4). Common tyramine-containing foods are bananas, pods of broad beans, avocado, aged cheese, chicken livers, yogurt, sour cream, and nuts.

Although some controversy still remains regarding mechanisms and the role of tyramine as a migraine precipitant, its avoidance usually is included in a comprehensive migraine treatment program.

Sodium Nitrite

Sodium nitrite is a food-coloring and preserving agent found in cured meats such as hot dogs, bacon, ham, and various processed meats and fish. The amounts added to foods are federally regulated because of possible carcinogenic properties. Small amounts can cause headaches in susceptible individuals by inducing vasodilation of cerebral blood vessels. The headache usually follows within one hour of ingestion.

Similar headaches sometimes are experienced in patients after taking nitrates, which are found in many anginal and vascular medications or vitamin supplements containing niacin or nicotinic acid.

Monosodium Glutamate (MSG)

MSG is a popular flavor enhancer and food preservative. It is commonly found in Chinese food, processed meats, frozen dinners, canned soups, soy sauce, and seasonings. Glutamic acid may have neuroexcitatory properties (2) and may interfere with glucose transport to the brain, resulting in cerebral vasodilation and, thus, vascular headache(s). Migraineurs who ingest MSG often experience a severe attack within hours of ingestion. However, some sufferers can ingest trace amounts with no apparent effect.

MSG can provoke the so-called "Chinese food syndrome" in nonmigrainous persons if taken in sufficient quantitites (as found in Chinese food). Symptoms can include headache, facial flushing, diaphoresis, mood disturbances, gastrointestinal (GI) distress, paresthesias, and chest pain. This susceptibility may be due to an inability to metabolize MSG properly (6).

Precipitating Causes of Migraine

Phenylethylamine

It has been known for many years that chocolate can precipitate migraine. It contains little tyramine, but does contain beta phenylethylamine, which is believed to be the provocative agent. Phenylethylamine is a potent vasoactive amine and also is found in some cheeses and red wine. The headache usually results within 12 hours of intake. It has been theorized by Sandler (7) that phenylethylamine releases vasoactive substances from the lungs that may have a secondary effect on the cerebral vasculature, resulting in vasodilation.

Alcohol

Alcohol is a nonspecific vasodilator that can provoke migraine attacks in susceptible individuals. It is thought to depress or alter central vasomotor centers, because the direct action of alcohol on blood vessels is insignificant (4). Of all the precipitating agents, alcohol most consistently provokes headaches in the largest number of patients.

Some migraine sufferers find that they can drink certain types of alcohol in small amounts, but not other types. This probably is due to the presence of vasoconstrictive compounds such as tyramine or histamine found in certain brands. The types more likely to induce headaches are red wines, brandy, and gin.

Overindulgence of alcohol often precipitates a migraine-like headache in nonsufferers and a prolonged migraine in sufferers. Interestingly, drinking alcohol in a relaxed environment, free of noise, smoke, snacks, and tension, may not trigger the hangover headache. This probably is due to relaxation and the absence of other triggering and aggravating factors.

Caffeine

Caffeine is a CNS stimulant that produces vascular constriction and is not a primary cause of headaches. Usually, caffeine is not a problem for most persons. However, excessive consumption of coffee, colas, or caffeine-containing analgesics may lead to a relative rebound vasodilation and headache, if consumption is suddenly reduced or delayed. Although this phenomenon can occur in many individuals, migraine sufferers seem to be particularly susceptible. As the last dose wears off, a headache may result, which is relieved by more caffeine or becomes more severe as caffeine is withheld. In some cases, individuals who consume significant amounts during the week may experience weekend headaches if intake is decreased. This caffeine deprivation also accounts for many headaches present on awakening.

Occasionally, patients will report the start of headaches shortly after the ingestion of minimal amounts of caffeine. Whether this is due to a true biological mechanism or the power of suggestion is difficult to determine. Many persons can consume up to 200 mg of caffeine per day without difficulty. However, one large mug of coffee can contain as much as 250 mg of caffeine (see Table 2).

Fasting

Skipping meals, prolonged fasting, or dieting can provoke migraine attacks in susceptible individuals. Five hours of fasting during waking hours and 13 hours of fasting overnight were shown to be provocative in a large survey of women sufferers (8). The mechanism is presumed to involve relative hypoglycemia, or lowering of blood sugar, which causes vasodilation. This hypoglycemic mechanism also has been suggested in studies by Dexter (9) and Blau (10).

Many migraine sufferers find that morning headaches occur when they sleep late on weekends or holidays. The same patients find that headaches do not occur if they arise at the usual time and eat something before returning to bed for extra sleep.

The fasting migraine can be prevented by eating regularly and avoiding any waking fasting for more than four hours. Meals should be well balanced with adequate protein, which digests more slowly than carbohydrates. Some patients who suffer from morning headaches or exercise headaches may benefit from protein snacks before going to bed or exercising.

TABLE 2 Sources of Caffeine

Coffee: 5-8-oz. cup	
drip	100-150 mg
percolated	65-125 mg
instant	40-110 mg
decaf-brewed	2-5 mg
decaf-instant	2 mg
Tea: 5-8-oz. cup	
bag, loose	20-75 mg
canned ice tea	25-35 mg
Soft drinks: 12-oz. glass	
cola	33-60 mg
Mountain Dew	54 mg
Dr. Pepper	38 mg
Chocolate	
bar, 1 oz.	3-6 mg
cocoa, 8 oz.	50 mg
bittersweet, 1 oz.	25-35 mg
Over-the-counter medication	
Excedrin	66 mg
Vanquish	60 mg
Anacin	32 mg
Midol	32 mg
Cope	32 mg

Other

Artificial sweeteners, in particular aspartame, have been implicated in precipitating migraine. Although some patients report more headaches with intake, investigative studies do not seem to support this theory.

Head pain of the temple, ear, forehead, or palate can be precipitated in susceptible individuals by ice cream. Cooling of the oral pharynx causes excessive vascular reaction, since many migraineurs demonstrate unstable vasomotor regulation. Raskin and Knittle (11) found that 93% of 59 migraineurs and 31% of 49 nonmigraineurs experienced headache after eating ice cream. My experience, though considerably less, is that a high percentage of migraineurs do report rapidly developing headache following the ingestion of ice cream or significantly cold foods.

Various other foods or additives that are thought to precipitate migraine attacks are reported by patients' physicians. The more commonly reported triggers are fats, milk products, various fruits and vegetables, and salt. Whether these represent true triggers or idiosyncratic reactions is yet to be determined.

HORMONAL INFLUENCES ON MIGRAINE

The influence of hormones on the migrainous patient is significant. The majority of migrainous sufferers are women, with increased headache problems occurring with menarche, menses, menopause, gynecologic irregularities, and while taking hormonal supplements or oral contraceptives. Adult women are subject to internal fluctuations of hormones during the menstrual cycle, which exert a significant effect on headache frequency and severity in many sufferers.

Supporting this relationship are other observations regarding migraine patients. The incidence of migraine in prepubescent boys and girls is about equal, suggesting no hereditary sex predilection. However, as girls undergo the adolescent maturing process, their incidence of migraine increases to more than double that of boys, and many migrainous boys experience only rare attacks after puberty.

Sixty percent of women seen by physicians for migraine headache report some relationship of their headaches to the menstrual cycle (12). Of this group of patients, as many as 25% may suffer with menstrual migraine (12) (headaches that occur exclusively with menses). The physiology of menstrually related migraine is not clearly understood at this time. However, it is believed to be related to the natural withdrawal of estrogen in the premenstrual phase of the menstrual cycle (13). Other mechanisms have been suggested, some of which are prostaglandin changes, fluid and glucose imbalances, and vitamin or immunologic deficiencies.

Precipitating Causes of Migraine

Oral Contraceptives

Migrainous women who use estrogen oral contraceptives often experience an increase in headache severity or frequency. This increase may occur immediately or many months after initiation of therapy. Some women without a migrainous history will develop migraine only after the beginning of oral contraception (14). The cessation of oral contraception may result in a decrease or improvement of attacks in some patients. However, in many patients, attacks may persist for extended periods of time. Occasionally, migrainous women will experience headache improvement with oral contraception.

Higher estrogen-dose birth-control pills seem to cause more of a problem than the lower dosed. Nonetheless, even those containing minimal estrogen can precipitate severe migraine attacks. During the month, the most vulnerable time for headache is the hormone-free period just before menstruation.

The risk of stroke in migrainous women taking oral contraceptives is increased. This is presumed to be due to an increased tendency for platelet aggregation and clot formation (15). Women who experience complicated migraine, whose attacks change in character, or who develop neurologic symptoms while taking oral contraceptives should discontinue their use.

Pregnancy

The majority of migrainous women experience significant headache improvement after the third month of pregnancy. The mechanism by which pregnancy causes migraine relief is not clear. The absence of cyclic rises and falls of estrogen levels, rising estrogenic hormones, changes in platelet aggregation, and protective secretions by the developing baby have been suggested.

I have conducted an extensive survey of female migraine sufferers who experience relief during pregnancy. Interviews and questionnaires were completed on sufferers and their mothers, grandmothers, and children when applicable. Results were inconclusive and did not suggest a consistent pattern of headache relief among the sufferers, parents, or siblings during pregnancy. However, those women who experienced significant headaches with menses and ovulation seemed to fare better during pregnancy.

Estrogen Replacement

Menopausal women and those having undergone hysterectomies who experience vasomotor symptoms often are treated with replacement estrogen. In general, estrogen therapy intensifies migraine and should be avoided whenever possible. If necessary, the synthetic form of estrogen may be of more benefit than the conjugated forms (16). Dosages should be kept as low as possible, and continuous therapy usually is more beneficial than interrupted therapy (17).

WEATHER

Weather changes seem to be obvious migraine precipitants to some sufferers. However, various studies do not support this theory. Instead, increased headaches tend to be related to the seasons, with spring and fall being the most difficult times for many sufferers (18).

Low barometric pressure that precedes a storm has long been associated with increased pain and illness. Severe winds throughout the world, such as the Santa Ana of Southern California, the Sharov of Israel, or the Foehn of Switzerland, are reported to cause illness and increased headache (19). Sulman (20) believed that internal physiologic changes occur as a result of high concentrations of atmospheric positive ions associated with such winds. These changes, characterized by increased serotonin levels, could be responsible for the early stages of migraine attacks.

ALTITUDE CHANGES

Headache is a consistent and prominent symptom of mountain or altitude sickness. Acute altitude sickness can occur in susceptible individuals exposed to altitudes of greater than 8,000 feet. It occurs in varying degrees and can include headache several hours after exposure, dyspnea, rapid pulse, anorexia, insomnia, mental disturbances, and pulmonary edema. The headache resembles migraine, is characterized by throbbing, and is aggravated by exertion, cough, movement, and lying down. It is presumed to be caused by relative hypoxia with reactive vasodilation and/or mild cerebral edema (21). Inhalation of oxygen, a gradual return to low altitude, cool fluids, and cautious use of ergotamine or isometheptene can be helpful in relieving the headache.

Migraine sufferers often report the precipitation of headache while traveling by airplane. Commercial airliners are reported to be pressurized to approximately 8,000 feet above sea level. However, the age and mechanical condition of the aircraft greatly affect the actual atmospheric pressure experienced by passengers. Whether exposure to increased altitude with relative hypoxia is the sole precipitating cause of the migraine attack is questionable.

External environmental factors are significant when traveling by air. There are important preflight stressors such as traffic, crowded airports, luggage difficulties, lines, and delays. During the flights, passengers are exposed to excessive flight noises and dry air, may become dehydrated, and often feel cramped. The combination of these factors and exposure to increased altitude often are enough to provoke a migraine attack in many individuals. Adequate hydration, relaxation techniques, exercise, and, in some cases, preflight medication, can be preventive.

At our center, in a recent blind study involving six migrainous patients who consistently experienced air-travel headache, attacks were decreased equally with diazepam or isometheptene as compared to placebo. Each of the six patients was pretreated with isometheptene 65 mg for two flights, diazepam 5 mg for two flights, and placebo for two flights. Pretreatment with isometheptene and diazepam decreased migraine attacks by 80%.

PSYCHOLOGICAL FACTORS

Personality traits such as perfectionism or a tendency to make too many self-imposed demands may increase the frequency of headaches in those persons already predisposed to migraine. Stressful events, both good and bad, or prolonged periods of stress can have a marked effect on the migraine sufferer. What actually constitutes stress varies tremendously from patient to patient. Simple changes in routine, changes in one's job, moving, family illness, or feuds are examples of frequently encountered stressful events. Many patients report that headaches occur after the stressful event or in the let-down period.

During major crises, such as a child suffering with a critical injury or illness, there is a notable absence of attacks. When the crisis has resolved, significant headaches often occur. Surprisingly, the same patient may find that rather minor stress, such as being late or a slight disagreement, may quickly precipitate severe attacks.

Depression can be a significant trigger of migraine headache (22). Many patients suppress anger and do not allow their true feelings to be expressed. This usually originates in childhood, when controlled good behavior was necessary to gain acceptance or promote family harmony (23). Migraineurs often rechannel their repressed hostilities into an ambitious quest for success. Continued suppression of true feelings can lead to significant conflict and depression.

EXERTION

Physical exercise or exertion such as sneezing, defecation, prolonged laughing, and sexual activity may precipitate a migrainous attack in susceptible individuals. The headache starts within minutes of the activity and may become severe immediately or progress gradually. Location of the pain is variable, and attacks can last from minutes to hours. Headaches induced by prolonged exertion usually are longer and more severe. The headaches may be prevented by pretreatment with medications, such as indomethacin, beta-blocking agents, ergotamine, or isometheptene, or by quantitative warm-up before strenuous exercise (24). Care should be taken with these patients to ensure that there is no organic problem causing the symptoms, though such problems are uncommon.

ENVIRONMENTAL

Many migraine sufferers are extremely sensitive to strong sensory stimuli and experience headache from various environmental sources. Bright lights, prolonged sun exposure, glare from water or snow, flickering lights, odors, and smoke commonly are reported to be precipitants. Sudden weather changes or prolonged exposure to the cold or heat also seem to increase patients' susceptibility to migraine attacks. These precipitating factors tend to be more significant for most patients during periods of stress or fatigue.

REFERENCES

1. Blau, J., and Diamond, S. (1985). Dietary factors in migraine precipitation: The physician's view, *Headache, 25*: 184-87.
2. Diamond, S., Prager, J., and Freitag, F. (1986). Diet and migraine, *Postgraduate Medicine, 79(4)*: 279-86.
3. Hanington, E., and Harper, A. (1968). The role of tyramine in the actiology of migraine and related studies on the cerebral and extracerebral circulation, *Headache, 8*: 84-96.
4. Diamond, S., and Dalessio, DJ. (1978). *Practicing Physician's Approach to Headaches* (2nd ed.), Williams & Williams, Baltimore, p. 55.
5. Krnjevic, K. (1974). Chemical nature of synoptic transmission in vertebrates, *Physical Review, 54*: 419.
6. Raskin, N. (1978). Hot dog, Chinese food, ice cream and cough headache. *Consultant*, 32-40.
7. Sandler, M., Youdin, M., and Hanington, E. (1974). A phenylethylamine oxidizing defect in migraine, *Nature, 250(464)*: 335-37.
8. Dalton, K. (1975). Food intake prior to migraine attacks. Study of 2313 spontaneous attacks, *Headache, 15*: 188-93.
9. Dexter, J., and Byer, J. (1981). The evaluation of 118 patients treated with low sucrose, frequent feeding diet, *Headache, 21*: 125.
10. Blau, S., and Pike, D. Effect of diabetes on migraine, *Lancet, 2*: 251-43.
11. Raskin, N., and Knittle, S. (1976). Ice cream headache and orthostatic symptoms in patients with migraine, *Headache, 16*: 22-25.
12. Horowski, R. (1976). Possible role of gonodal hormones as triggering factors in migraine, *Functional Neurology, 1*: 405-14.

13. Somerville, B. (1972). The role of estradiol withdrawal in the etiology of menstrual migraine headache, *Neurology, 22*: 355-65.
14. Blau, J. (ed.). (1987). *Migraine Clinical and research aspects*, John Hopkins University Press, Baltimore, p. 467.
15. Irez, N., McAllister, H., and Henry, S. (1978). Oral contraceptives and stroke in young women; a clinical pathological correlation, *Neurology, 28*: 1216-19.
16. Raskin, N. (1988). *Headache*, Churchill Livingstone, New York, p. 55.
17. Kudrow, L. (1975). The relationshipo of headache frequency to hormone use in migraine, *Headache, 15*: 36-40.
18. Heyck, H. (1981). *Headache and Facial Pain,* Year Book Medical Publishers Chicago, p. 45.
19. Raskin, N. (1988). *Headache* (2nd ed.), Churchill Livingstone, New York, p. 57.
20. Sulman, F. (1971). "Migraine in Climatic Heart Stress, Its Prophylaxis and Treatment," Proceedings of International Headache Symposium, Elsinore, Denmark.
21. Appenzeller, O. (1978). Cerebrovascular aspects of headache, *Medical Clinics of North America, 62*: 474.
22. Lambert, R., and Burnet, D. (1985). Prevention of exercise induced migraine by quantitative warm-up, *Headache, 25*: 317-19.
23. Diamond, S., and Diamond-Falk, J. (1982). *Advice from the Diamond Headache Clinic*, International Universities Press, New York, p. 89.
24. Adler, C., Adler, S., and Packard, R. (1987). *Psychiatric Aspects of Headache*, Williams & Wilkins, Baltimore, p. 171.

3

Abortive Treatment of Migraine

Robert S. Kunkel *Cleveland Clinic Foundation, Cleveland, Ohio*

INTRODUCTION

In treating the person with migraine, it is important to help the individual to identify and avoid trigger factors, as discussed in other areas of this book. Prophylactic agents, if indicated, may reduce the frequency of attacks, but rarely eliminate all attacks. As a result, most individuals on prophylactic therapy also wlll need to have abortive therapy for their acute migraine attacks. Patients with infrequent attacks should be treated only with abortive agents and should not be given daily preventive medications. An exception would be infrequent but prolonged attacks not responding to abortive therapy.

Attacks of migraine with aura (classic migraine) and migraine without aura (common migraine) are treated in the same manner. If the aura is prolonged and severe, it probably is wise to avoid vasoconstrictive agents, although there has been no positive evidence of any detrimental effect of these drugs when used in proper dosages. In patients with prolonged visual or neurologic prodromal symptoms or in patients having aura without headache (migraine equivalents, acephalgic migraine), vasodilating agents may be useful.

NONPHARMACOLOGIC THERAPY

There are some nonpharmacologic treatments that patients occasionally find helpful for the acute attack. Cold packs applied to the scalp, along with pressure, may help to reduce the pulsating pain. Some patients will find black coffee helpful early in the attack. A dark, quiet environment and sleep will help most migraine attacks. The City Migraine Clinic in London has had success in treating acute migraine attacks with rest, antinauseants, and simple analgesics such as aspirin or acetaminophen.

Electrical stimulation, such as that induced by the usual TENS unit, has not proven to be very helpful in acute migraine. Further development and refinement of such devices continues, and several devices specifically designed for use in headache are available. Early reports are encouraging, and clinical trials are under way. Other therapies that have been promoted, such as hot and cold showers and the use of pressure points, are unreliable.

VASOCONSTRICTIVE AGENTS

Ergotamine tartrate has been the drug of choice for treating the acute migraine attack for many years. It is a vasoconstrictive agent that predominantly affects the carotid system. Ergotamine tartrate also is a serotonin antagonist; sensitizes smooth muscle to sympathetic stimulation; inhibits free uptake of monoamines, and, in moderate doses, stimulates alpha adrenocepters (1). All of these actions probably contribute to its effectiveness in the acute migraine attack.

Contraindications to the use of ergotamine include evidence of sepsis or other systemic illness, local infection, liver disease, or vascular disease. Ergotamine tartrate should be used with caution

Abortive Treatment of Migraine

in persons with hypertension or peptic ulcer disease. Toxic effects such as paresthesias, muscle cramps, and ischemic changes in organs or limbs will occur rarely. These problems usually arise with the use of large dosages; occasionally, however, there are persons with marked sensitivity to ergotamine in whom these toxic effects will occur with a very small dosage. Gastrointestinal symptoms such as nausea, vomiting, abdominal pain, and diarrhea are not uncommon side effects of ergotamine administration. These adverse effects may occur with small amounts and are not necessarily related to the dosage administered.

Ergotamine tartrate is available as an oral or sublingual tablet, rectal suppository, inhalant, or parenteral injection. It is most effective when taken early in the attack and, in general, should be used as soon as the patient realizes that an attack is coming. Patients with a specific aura should take ergotamine at the onset of the aura.

The oral tablets are most widely used in the United States. All oral and rectal preparations of ergotamine tartrate, except Bellergal®, contain 100 mg of caffeine. Pentobarbital sodium and levorotatory alkaloids of belladonna also are present in some tablets and rectal suppositories. The ergotamine medihaler, the sublingual tablets, and parenteral dihydroergotamine do not contain caffeine, belladonna, or pentobarbital. The most effective nonparenteral form is the rectal suppository, which is readily absorbed even when there may be severe nausea and vomiting present. Diarrhea, which is not uncommon in the migraine attack, will limit the suppository's usefulness. The inconvenience of its use also is a limiting factor.

The usual dosage of oral ergotamine tartrate is two tablets (1 mg of ergotamine each) at the onset of the aura or the pain, followed by one tablet every half hour for two or three additional doses if necessary. If this amount does not break the attack, more ergotamine is unlikely to help and will only increase the number of side effects. The rectal suppository (2 mg of ergotamine tartrate) is used at the onset of the attack and followed by another suppository in one hour if needed. Many patients will find that one-half or even one-third of a suppository is effective and will, in

TABLE 1 Abortive Therapy for Migraine Attacks

Preparation	Dosage
Vasoconstrictor agents	
Ergotamine tartrate	
oral: Cafergot®, Cafergot PB®, Wigraine®	Two at onset; one every ½ hour X 3 PRN*
rectal: Cafergot®, Cafergot PB®, Wigraine®	One at onset; one in 1 hr PRN
sublingual: ergostat®, Ergomar®, Wigrettes®	One at onset; one in 1 hr PRN
IM or IV: dihydroergotamine (DHE-45)	One puff at onset; repeat in 5 min
Isometheptene mucate	
oral: Midrin®, Migralam®	Two at onset; two in 1 hr PRN
Anti-inflammatory agents	
Nonsteroidal	
Meclofenamate sodium (Meclomen®)	100-200 mg at onset; repeat 1 hr PRN
Ibuprofen (Rufen®, Motrin®)	400-800 mg at onset; repeat 4 hrs PRN
Naproxen sodium (Anaprox®)	275-550 mg at onset; repeat 4 hrs PRN
Steroids	
Depo-Medrol®	40-80 mg IM†
Decadron-LA®	8-12 mg IM
Antiemetics	
Metoclopramide (Reglan®)	20 mg prior to abortive drug
Phenothiazines (promethazine, chlorpromazine, prochlorperazine)	Variable; oral, parenteral, rectal
Hydroxyzine pamoate (Atarax®, Vistaril®)	25-50 mg oral, parenteral

*As needed.
†Intramuscularly.

Abortive Treatment of Migraine 49

turn, reduce the number of side effects. An additional benefit of using a suppository is the fact that the patient usually has to lie down for 20 to 30 minutes and this, in itself, may be beneficial.

The sublingual tablet (2 mg of ergotamine tartrate) is placed under the tongue and repeated in one-half hour if necessary. The very unpleasant taste of the sublingual tablets makes them unacceptable to many patients. One puff of the inhalant form (0.36 mg of ergotamine tartrate) is used at the onset of the attack and repeated in five minutes, up to a total of six separate inhalations if necessary. The total amount of ergotamine tartrate should be limited to 6 mg in 24 hours and 12 mg in one week. At least 48 hours should elapse between courses of ergotamine tartrate to avoid the development of an ergotamine-rebound state.

The only parenteral form of ergotamine in the United States at this time is dihydroergotamine mesylate (DHE-45). It can be used intramuscularly or intravenously. One milligram given intramuscularly at hourly intervals to a total of 3 mg if needed is the recommended dosage. Once a specific dosage is found that aborts the attack, that amount may be given as a single dose if desired. Occasionally, DHE-45 may be given intravenously. One milligram should be given very slowly. Many physicians in the office setting or in the emergency room will use dihydroergotamine parenterally before resorting to the usual parenteral narcotics to treat an acute migraine attack. Dihydroergotamine, unlike ergotamine tartrate, often will abort an attack even if it has been going on for some time. This may alleviate the need for narcotics. Gastrointestinal side effects are less common with DHE-45 than with ergotamine tartrate.

Isometheptene mucate is the only other vasoconstrictive agent currently available for the treatment of acute migraine. It is available in a form combined with dichloralphenazone and acetaminophen and in a form combined with caffeine and acetaminophen. Isometheptene mucate is a sympathomimetic amine that constricts dilated vessels. Dichloralphenazone is a mild, nonbarbiturate sedative.

Isometheptene mucate is well tolerated and, although not as effective as ergotamine tartrate, often works quite well. The dosage is two capsules at the onset of headache symptoms, followed by one or two more capsules in an hour if necessary. One capsule can be repeated hourly for two or three more doses. It is recommended that the daily dosage be limited to eight capsules. Contraindications to the use of isometheptene mucate include glaucoma, severe renal or liver disease, and use with an MAO-inhibitor antidepressant. Isometheptene is not known to cause rebound headache even when used frequently

ERGOTAMINE-REBOUND HEADACHE

A serious problem with the use of ergotamine that seems to be seen with increasing frequency is rebound headache (2,3). It is well documented that frequent (daily or every other day) usage of ergotamine tartrate can lead to a recurring vascular headache that is stopped by use of ergotamine, only to recur 12 to 48 hours after dosing. The caffeine and barbiturate present in many ergotamine preparations also may be a factor in the rebound headache that develops. A vascular type of headache occurring at fairly regular intervals and responding to ergotamine tartrate should raise one's suspicions that a rebound or withdrawal situation exists.

The cause of ergotamine-rebound headache is unknown. It is postulated that this phenomenon occurs because of sensitization of blood-vessel walls and effects on the central nervous system. Disturbances in hypothalamic function and sympathetic control may be important factors (2).

It is recommended that a two- to three-day period of time elapse between courses of ergotamine tartrate to avoid the development of ergotamine-rebound headache. The total amount of ergotamine tartrate used for any one headache does not seem to be a factor, while the frequency of the drug's administration does.

The treatment of ergotamine-rebound headache is withdrawal from the drug. At times, this can be done by the patient with the help of analgesics and antiemetics to control the withdrawal symptoms. Recently, it has been reported (4) that the use of naproxen will help to reduce the symptoms during ergotamine withdrawal. Many persons dependent on ergotamine will need to

Abortive Treatment of Migraine

be hospitalized to accomplish the withdrawal successfully. Intravenous fluids, sedation, antiemetics, analgesics, and corticosteroids all may be necessary to help control the withdrawal symptoms.

ANALGESICS

Some patients with migraine may get relief with simple analgesics. Aspirin seems to be much more effective than acetaminophen for vascular headaches. Most patients with migraine, however, find that aspirin and acetaminophen are not very helpful in aborting attacks. Nonsteroidal anti-inflammatory drugs (NSAIDs) are being used more often for migraine. The exact mechanism by which these agents alleviate pain and control migraine is unknown. Their blocking of prostaglandin syntheses is probably most important.

The fast-acting NSAIDs such as meclofenamate sodium, ibuprofen, and naproxen sodium are all effective agents. Meclofenamate is the most rapidly absorbed and is effective and well tolerated. Occasionally, upper GI symptoms or diarrhea will occur. The usual dosage is 200 mg at the onset of the migraine attack, followed by 100 or 200 mg in one hour if necessary.

The nonsteroidal agents are a good choice when ergotamine is contraindicated, not tolerated, or ineffective. The nonsteroidals are contraindicated in persons with ulcer disease and should be used with caution in hypertensive patients. If used on a frequent basis, a patient's renal function needs to be monitored.

Simple analgesics, such as aspirin and acetaminophen, combined with barbiturates and caffeine, are widely prescribed for migraine. This type of combination often will be effective. To avoid the development of dependency, these analgesics should not be used frequently. Other analgesics such as codeine, propoxyphene hydrochloride (HCl) (Darvon®), and stronger agents such as oxycodone HCl (Percodan®), meperidine HCl (Demerol®), or hydromorphone HCl (Dilaudid®) may be useful and are acceptable if used infrequently. Meperidine hydrochloride is much less effective orally than when given as an intramuscular injection. For many migraine sufferers, nausea and vomiting make oral agents useless. Meperidine hydrochloride given by injection along with an antinauseant/sedative such as hydroxyzine pamoate or promethazine hydrochloride has become the standard parenteral therapy for an acute migraine attack that has not responded to oral agents.

SEDATIVES AND ANTIEMETICS

Sleep will be of benefit to most individuals having a migraine attack. Sedative drugs often are a useful adjunct in the treatment of acute migraine. Often, they are used along with analgesics or narcotics. Hydroxyzine pamoate and promethazine HCl 25 to 50 mg given intramuscularly are the most widely used. Either one also may be given by the oral or rectal route. Intravenous chlorpromazine used in the emergency room has been reported to be very effective in the acute migraine attack (5).

Many of the sedatives are also antiemetics. Hydroxyzine pamoate, promethazine HCl, and chlorpromazine all are useful for the nausea of migraine. Trimethobenzamide HCl (Tigan®) and metoclopramide HCl (Reglan®) cause little sedation. Metoclopramide HCl 10 to 20 mg given orally is a very effective antiemetic and has been shown to enhance the absorption and, therefore, the effectiveness of oral medication. It promotes gastric emptying by reducing the gastric atony and stasis that often occur in migraine (6). It acts peripherally as a cholinomimetic and centrally as a dopamine antagonist. It also can be given intravenously if desired. In patients with prominent nausea accompanying the migraine attack, metoclopramide should be given 15 to 20 minutes before using an oral vasoconstrictive agent or analgesic. Occasionally, metoclopramide will cause nervousness and tremor.

CORTICOSTEROIDS

Corticosteroids are useful in acute migraine. Oral or intramuscular steroids may be used. They do not act quickly, but often will bring an attack to an end within 12 to 24 hours. Their effectiveness probably is due to the fact that a sterile inflammation surrounding the extracranial vessels develops during the migraine

Abortive Treatment of Migraine

attack. This inflammation contributes to the pain. Methylprednisolone acetate (Depo-Medrol®) 40 to 80 mg or dexamethasone acetate (Decadron-LA®) 12 to 16 mg are given intramuscularly. At times, oral corticosteroids also will help when used for a few days. Forty to sixty milligrams of Prednisone® or its equivalent is used the first day and then rapidly tapered off over three to five days. Corticosteroids are most widely used in status migrainosus.

STATUS MIGRAINOSUS

When a migraine attack lasts more than three days because it has not responded to the usual abortive agents, it is termed *status migrainosus*. Such intractable migraine usually warrants parenteral therapy (7). Most patients with status migrainosus have used excessive ergotamine and analgesics, which may add to the perpetuation of the migraine attack. Sedation, along with corticosteroids and antinauseants, usually will help (8). Corticosteroids given intramuscularly are a very important part of the treatment of a prolonged migraine siege. Dexamethasone acetate 12 to 16 mg or methylprednisolone acetate 40 to 80 mg are the usual agents used. In addition, sedation, narcotics, and antiemetics often will be necessary. Dihydroergotamine mesylate injection (DHE-45) 1 mg intravenously every eight hours for three to five doses may be very effective in breaking up an intractable migraine. Raskin (9) reported good results when combining intravenous DHE-45 and metoclopramide 10 mg given intravenously every eight hours for two days. Within 48 hours, 49 of 55 patients so treated became headache-free. It is of interest that the DHE-45 seemed to be quite effective even though the headache had been present for days or even weeks.

AURA WITHOUT HEADACHE (MIGRAINE EQUIVALENTS)

Some patients will have visual and/or neurological symptoms without any headache phase. If these spells occur quite frequently, prophylactic medication is indicated. The same prophylactic medications used for migraine will be effective. Most patients, however, do not have these attacks often enough to warrant daily prophylactic therapy. If the attacks are disturbing, abortive therapy is indicated. Ergotamine tartrate has been used for years and may shorten the symptoms, but many physicians hesitate to recommend a vasoconstrictive agent for these symptoms, which may be due in part to vasoconstriction. Early studies by Wolff and his workers showed prompt but transient relief of the visual symptoms of migraine with amyl nitrate inhalation (10). Carbon dioxide and oxygen also cleared these symptoms.

Nifedipine sublingually has been reported to promptly abort the visual and neurological symptoms of migraine (11,12). Visual symptoms may be aborted promptly by isoproterenol inhalation (13). Nitroglycerin used sublingually also will promptly clear visual and neurologic symptoms in many patients. If used early in the attack, most patients do not have an exacerbation of the headache (14).

SUMMARY

All patients who have migraine will need to have treatment for their acute attacks whether or not they are on daily prophylactic medication. There is a wide range of pharmacologic agents available for the physician to prescribe. Underlying conditions may dictate which abortive agents can be used in any one patient.

REFERENCES

1. Tfelt-Hansen, P. (1986). The effect of ergotamine on the arterial system in man, *Acta Pharm. et Toxi., 59*(*suppl. III*):
2. Saper, J. R., and Jones, J. M. (1986). Ergotamine tartrate dependency: Features and possible mechanisms, *Clin. Neuropharm., 9*: 244-256.
3. Tfelt-Hansen, P. and Krabbe, A. E. (1981). Ergotamine abuse: Do patients benefit from withdrawal? *Cephal., 1*: 29-32.
4. Mathew, N. T. (1987). Amelioration of ergotamine withdrawal symptoms with naproxen, *Headache, 27*: 130-133.

5. Lane, P. L. and Ross, R. (1985). Intravenous chlorpromazine—preliminary results in acute migraine, *Headache, 25*: 302-304.
6. Volans, G. N. (1978). Migraine and drug absorption, *Clin. Pharmacokinetics, 3*: 313-318.
7. Couch, J. R. and Diamond S. (1983). Status migrainosus: Causative and therapeutic aspects, *Headache, 23*: 94-101.
8. Gallagher, R. M. (1986). Emergency treatment of intractable migraine, *Headache, 26*: 74-75.
9. Raskin, N. H. (1986). Repetitive intravenous dihydroergotamine as therapy for intractable migraine, *Neurol., 36*: 995-997.
10. Dalessio, D. J., ed. (1980). *Wolff's Headache and Other Head Pain* (4th ed.), Oxford University Press, New York, pp. 71-74.
11. Miller, F. W. and Santoro, T. J. (1984). Nifedipine in the treatment of migraine headache and amaurosis fugax in patients with systemic lupus erythematosus, *NEJM, 311*: 921.
12. Tucker, R. M. (1984). Sublingual nifedipine relieves migraine prodromes, *Headache, 24*: 285.
13. Kupersmith, M. J., Hass, W. K., and Chase, N. E. (1979). Isoproterenol treatment of visual symptoms in migraine, *Stroke, 10*: 299-305.
14. Kunkel, R. S. (1982). Vasodilator therapy for classic migraine headache, *Advances in Migraine Research and Therapy* (F. C. Rose, ed.), Raven Press, New York, pp. 205-209.

4

The Use of Beta Blockers in Migraine

Frederick G. Freitag *Diamond Headache Clinic, Ltd., and University of Chicago, Chicago, Illinois*

INTRODUCTION

The beta-adrenergic-blocking agents have gained a prominent role in the treatment of migraine headaches over the past 20 years. With the exception of ergots, these are the only other agents approved for the treatment of migraine headache in the United States by the Food and Drug Administration (FDA). In this chapter, I will review some of the pharmacologic aspects of this group of agents, especially as they pertain to the treatment of migraine. Also, I will discuss studies of the various beta blockers, as they are more commonly referred to, in the treatment of migraine headache.

PHARMACOLOGY

The beta-adrenergic-blocking drugs possess a variety of pharmacologic actions that may play an important role in understanding the potential mechanism of action in migraine prophylaxis. All of these agents, by definition, exert an antagonizing effect on the beta adrenoceptors (1), which may be subdivided into the beta-1 and beta-2 subtypes (2). In addition, certain beta-adrenergic antagonists also may have an agonizing effect, possibly incomplete, on these same receptors. This partial agonist effect also has been termed *intrinsic sympathomimetic activity*. The beta blockers also may act as potent antagonists of 5-hydroxytryptamine, also known as serotonin (3). Additional properties of the beta-adrenergic-blocking agents also have been evaluated for their potential role in influencing the efficacy of certain beta blockers as compared to other agents in the prophylaxis of migraine (4). These characteristics, which Shanks considered, included lipophylicity versus hydrophilicity and membrane-stabilizing activity. Other researchers (5,6) have examined the cerebral circulation effects of beta-adrenergic blockers and the relationship of muscle-nerve sympathetic activity as it pertains to migraine treatment (7). Schoenen (8) and colleagues (9) examined the role of the central sympathetic system in migraine and the role of beta blockers in influencing it. Because platelets have been implicated in migraine, the effect of beta blockade on the platelets has been studied (10, 11). The role played by blood levels of beta blockers in influencing migraine treatment also has been studied (12-14).

BETA SUBTYPE SELECTIVITY

The vast majority of beta-adrenergic-blocking agents are not selective in binding to either the beta-1 or beta-2 subtype receptors. The assessment of the beta-2 adrenergic-blocking effect may be studied by measurement of peripheral vascular resistance response to infusion of epinephrine. The beta-1 adrenergic-blocking effect may be studied by maximal treadmill exercise heart rates (15). Of those agents tested in migraine prophylaxis, only atenolol, metoprolol, and, possibly, acebutol are selective for the beta-1 receptors, at usual dosages. This action provides a cardioselective property that avoids the effects on bronchial and peripheral beta-2 receptors. Although this action may be advantageous in the overall

The Use of Beta Blockers in Migraine

consideration of beta-blocker therapy, it does not correlate with effectiveness in migraine treatment. Two of these beta-1 selective agents, atenolol and metoprolol, have been shown to be beneficial in migraine prophylaxis, as have several nonselective beta-adrenoceptor-blocking agents. Recently interest has increased in the use of beta-2 selective blocking agents (ICI 115, 551) in migraine prophylaxis. However, long-term safety concerns with these agents, based on animal-model studies, forced termination of the study (16).

PARTIAL AGONIST ACTIVITY

Certain beta-blocking agents—specifically, alprenolol, oxprenolol, pindolol, and acebutolol—are known to exert antagonistic effects on beta-1 and, in most cases, beta-2 receptors. These agents also have been demonstrated to possess an agonizing effect on these same receptors. This effect is manifested by less reduction in heart rate and cardiac output, as well as by a decrease in peripheral resistance, as compared to those beta-blocking agents devoid of the partial agonist activity. Correlation of the presence of partial agonist activity in a beta-blocking agent with the efficacy to prevent migraine reveals that those agents possessing this activity are not beneficial in migraine therapy.

SEROTONIN ANTAGONISTIC EFFECTS

The neurotransmitter 5-hydroxytryptamine, which also is found in the peripheral vascular system, has been linked to migraine and other headache disorders. Several potent antagonists of serotonin have proven useful in the prophylaxis of migraine. These agents include methysergide, cyproheptadine, and amitriptyline, which are discussed in other chapters. Several beta blockers, such as propranolol and oxprenolol, have demonstrated strong antagonizing actions on 5-hydroxytryptamine. Of these, only propranolol exerts positive effects in migraine prevention. While oxprenolol is inactive in migraine, it does have serotonin-antagonizing effects.

Antenolol has little affinity for serotonin receptors, but has shown good results in migraine treatment.

CENTRAL NERVOUS SYSTEM PENETRATION

A good correlation exists between the relative degree of lipid solubility of beta-blocking agents and their ability to penetrate the central nervous system (17). Those agents with the highest lipid-soluble properties can more readily penetrate the blood-brain barrier. In reviewing this lipid solubility and the correlating penetration of the central nervous system, a good correlation with exerting significant prophylactic effects in migraine is not shown. Two of the more hydrophilic agents, nadolol and atenolol, produce little CNS effect, yet are beneficial in migraine. By contrast, the other beta blockers are lipophilic and, of these, only propranolol, timolol, and metoprolol have been shown to be beneficial in migraine treatment

MEMBRANE-STABILIZING ACTIVITY

The membrane-stabilizing activity of certain beta blockers occurs on peripheral nerve cells and in the heart. From a therapeutic viewpoint, it is important to note that those beta blockers possessing this action have antiarrhythmic effects attributed to the class I antiarrhythmics. However, no direct connection exists between beta blockers that possess this activity and those that do not, and their efficacy in migraine. Although propranolol and metoprolol possess membrane-stabilizing activity and nadolol and atenolol do not, all four have demonstrated beneficial effects in migraine therapy.

CEREBRAL CIRCULATION

Edvinsson (6) has examined in vitro models, using both animal and human pial arteries, of the beta-adrenergic receptors and their response to beta-blocking agents. In a study of feline intracranial

The Use of Beta Blockers in Migraine

and extracranial arteries, the effect of four vasoactive amines—isoproterenol, adrenaline, noradrenaline, and terbutaline—was to dilate tonically contracted vessels, and the study demonstrated that the intracranial arteries were mediated by beta-1 receptors. Furthermore, propranolol antagonized this effect on both vascular sources, as would be expected, based on its nonselective beta-adrenergic-receptor characteristics. A similar situation exists in rat cerebral arteries, where the effect of isoproterenol was blocked by the beta-1 selective antagonist, metoprolol. However, in human pial arteries, this action of metoprolol to antagonize isoproterenol was seen only to a varying degree, suggestive of both a beta-1 and beta-2 adrenergic-receptor mediaton of this process.

Olesen (5) examined the changes in cerebral circulation in patients undergoing carotid angiograms. Patients were injected with noradrenaline, adrenaline, isoprenaline, propranolol, or hydergine, and the effect on cerebral circulation was measured. Cerebral blood flow was measured with intra-arterial injection of xenon^{133}, and regional cerebral blood flow was measured with either a 16- or 35-point detector. After correction for $PACO_2$ and consideration of autoregulatory effects, there was little change with any of the injections, other than a 4% reduction in regional cerebral blood flow with propranolol, which was considered a central depressant response. Olesen concluded that the effects of propranolol on migraine were mediated by mechanisms other than an effect on cerebral blood vessels or regional cerebral blood flow.

AUTONOMIC DYSREGULATION

The alterations in cerebral blood flow that have been associated with migraine, and the tendency for migraineurs to experience Raynaud-like phenomena such as cold hands and feet, may represent a more generalized disturbance of autonomic function. Fagius and colleagues (7) studied the muscle-nerve sympathetic activity both in hypertensive patients treated with metoprolol and in a group of migraine patients during a migraine attack and in a headache-free period. Metoprolol was demonstrated to reduce the muscle-nerve sympathetic activity in hypertensive patients following long-term treatment. These researchers then examined a group of seven migraineurs and found that, during the headache-free intervals, the level of muscle-nerve sympathetic activity was similar to that of the nonmigraine patients. Additionally, no essential change in this measure of activity during attacks as compared to headache-free periods was noted in these seven patients. Fagius et al. (7) concluded that migraine is not a generalized sympathetic-system vasomotor disorder.

Jay and his associates (18) assessed the effect of the beta-adrenergic-blocking agent, propranolol, on the ability of migraine patients to learn vascular biofeedback training. In this study, the rapidity with which migraine patients were able to master biofeedback techniques was reduced in those patients using propranolol, versus those on no medications. However, the migraine patients on the beta blocker overall were able to develop similar skills with this technique, as compared to untreated patients. Understanding of biofeedback techniques was slowed in patients using electromyographic biofeedback for muscle-contraction headache and concomitantly using amitriptyline.

CENTRAL CATECHOLAMINE ACTIONS

Schoenen (8) has examined the central catecholaminergic system using contingent negative variation. This tool uses the electroencephalographic (EEG) recording of event-related slow cerebral potentials through an averaging device, while the patient performs a simple reaction-time task. Additionally, Schoenen cites the correlation of contingent-negative-variation differences in migraine patients as compared both to patients with tension headache and to control groups. Several groups of patients have been studied. In a retrospective study using metoprolol 50 mg, DeNoordhout and his colleagues (9) demonstrated a reduction of the contingent-negative-variation amplitude from a baseline comparable to untreated migraine control patients and a control group of nonheadache patients who underwent contingent-negative-variation trials on several occasions. In three of these patients, the result was seen as early in treatment as two weeks, suggesting a direct drug-related effect as opposed to an effect resulting from a decrease in the overall frequency of the migraine attacks over the three-month trial period.

A retrospective study also was conducted on patients who had been treated with either metoprolol or proparanolol. The study assessed the degree of success of these beta blockers in reducing the frequency of the headaches and also assessed the pretreatment contingent-negative-variation amplitude. The results suggested that the greater the degree of amplitude with this parameter in pretreatment, the greater the likelihood of successfully reducing migraine attacks. These results were compared to those of patients treated in a similar manner with the calcium-channel-entry blocker, flunarazine. In the flunarazine group, successful resolution of the migraines did not correlate with a normalization of the contingent-negative-variation amplitude. Although these studies suggest a useful role for contingent negative variation in both the study of migraine and the prediction of treatment outcome with beta blockers, the possibility of other factors being involved in migraine also is demonstrated.

PLATELET STUDIES

Two independently performed studies (10,11) examined the effect of the nonselective beta blocker, propranolol, and the selective beta-adrenergic antagonist, metoprolol, in migraine patients. Although neither study specifically examined the outcome effect of these agents, both studies evaluated the effect of these agents on platelet function. Some researchers have hypothesized that platelet function plays a role in the genesis of migraine. The studies by Joseph's group and Hedman's group assessed the changes in adenosine diphosphate (ADP)-induced platelet aggregation and platelet secretion as measured by adenosine triphosphate (ATP) release. Both groups used standard treatment dosages of these agents—propranolol 40 mg twice a day (BID), metoprolol 50 mg BID. In each study, propranolol increased platelet aggregation and increased the platelet-release response. However, metoprolol produced either little change or a decrease in these two parameters. The conclusions reached by both groups suggested either that migraine is unrelated to platelet function or that the mechanism by which beta-adrenergic-blocking agents are effective in migraine is unrelated to platelet function.

PLASMA LEVELS

Several studies have been undertaken that attempted to correlate the plasma levels of propranolol and one of its metabolites, 4-hydroxypropranolol, and the clinical outcome in migraine patients. Kuritzky et al. (12) studied 26 patients treated with propranolol dosages of 80 mg to 240 mg per day in divided doses for at least three weeks. Sixty percent of their patients demonstrated a positive response to treatment, with a reduction in the frequency of the migraine attacks. The blood levels of propranolol varied from 1 to 79 ng/ml at 10 hours after the last oral dose to as high as 7 to 218 ng/ml at 2 hours after a dose of propranolol. No correlation was demonstrated between the plasma levels of propranolol and the reduction in the migraines. However, a correlation was noted among slowing of the standing pulse rate, beta-adrenergic blockade, and reduction in headache frequency. Similar correlations were found for headache severity and associated symptoms with decreases in parameters such as pulse rate and blood pressure.

Similarly, Cortelli and his colleagues (13), in a study of 22 patients treated with propranolol 40 to 240 mg per day in divided doses, failed to find a correlation between successful resolution of the migraines and plasma levels of propranolol, 4-hydroxypropranolol, or the sum of the two plasma levels. In contrast to Kuritzky's group (12), Cortelli's group failed to find a correlation between reduction in heart rate or beta blockade and improvement of migraine.

An interesting aspect of plasma levels was demonstrated by Gengo and associates (14). They described a patient who had achieved partial resolution of migraine except during the premenstrual phase of the menstrual cycle. Plasma propranolol levels demonstrated a significant reduction during this phase, although medication dosages were constant. This incident may partially explain the tendency for migraine to occur at menses in those female migraineurs whose attacks are controlled with beta-adrenergic-blocking agents. Additional controlled studies will be necessary to fully assess these therapeutic problems.

PHARMACOLOGIC SUMMARY

The beta-adrenergic-blocking drugs consist of a diverse group of agents that have significant variations in pharmacologic action. A review of these various actions attributes the effectiveness of a beta-adrenergic-blocking agent in migraine to the absence of partial agonistic activity. However, there are other pharmacologic considerations that are potentially important in selecting an agent, but that probably will have little effect on the final result of therapy.

Many pharmacologic characteristics are associated with the various beta-adrenergic blockers. Also, many hypotheses have been advanced on the etiology of migraine, and several attempts have been made to correlate the action of the proven migraine prophylactic beta blockers with the different hypotheses. In general, these studies have failed to provide useful correlations. The studies of contingent-negative-variation amplitude, and the possibility of predicting a successful outcome in migraine treatment, did not offer much insight into the pathogenesis of migraine. However, these studies may prove helpful in selecting a pharmacologic agent for migraine therapy.

Studies of Beta-Adrenergic-Blocking Agents in Migraine Prophylaxis

The literature contains diverse reports on the role of beta-adrenergic-blocking agents in migraine prophylaxis. Like reports on other classes of therapeutic agents, these reports often develop as scattered case reports, followed by open trials of the agent, thus leading to double-blind studies comparing the therapeutic agent to placebo or another therapeutic agent. In those double-blind studies, a specific therapeutic agent may be compared to an agent from a different pharamacologic class that has been demonstrated as effective on the indication being tested. Alternatively, two agents with similar pharmacologic effects may be assessed to determine which agent will be established as a therapeutic tool. Eventually, newer agents are compared to assess their effectiveness for a similar outcome, but through another mechanism of action. This evolutionary process of drug research and development is well exemplified by the beta-adrenergic-blocking agents.

Case Reports and Open Studies
Propranolol

In 1968, Wykes (19) reported on four patients with histories of concomitant angina pectoris and migraine headaches. Both disorders improved with initiation of propranolol treatment for angina pectoris. Within a few months, several case reports were published. Behes and his associates (20) reported on patients with extra systoles and migraine, and Hall (21) described patients with hypertrophic cardiomyopathy and migraine. In these patients, propranolol was used to treat the cardiac disease and subsequently alleviated the migraine headaches.

These case reports of successful migraine prophylaxis with propranolol were reported by Sales and Bada (22) in an open trial of the beta-1 selective agent, practolol, in 44 patients with common migraine, typical migraine, or histaminic cephalgia. A good response to this agent was reported by 39 patients. In 1980, Ljung (23) reported that metoprolol was beneficial in three patients with migraine headache.

In 1974, Wideroe and Vigander (24) enrolled 49 patients into an open-label trial of propranolol in migraine prophylaxis. The patients were given 160 mg daily of propranolol for six months. In the initial phase of the study, 84% of the patients had an excellent response, and an additional 6 (12%) had at least a partial improvement in their migraine attacks. Subsequently, 30 of these patients were enrolled in a double-blind, placebo-controlled, crossover study with two phases of treatment that lasted three months. The study was completed by 26 patients. Propranolol was preferred to placebo by 21 patients and the 5 remaining patients denied preference for either treatment. The attack frequency decreased from 1.7 during placebo treatment to 0.4 during propranolol treatment.

Nair (25) subsequently reported that 80 mg per day of propranolol was effective in migraine prophylaxis. In his study, 20 patients who had been taking and continued to be treated with 15 mg per day of prochlorperazine were treated with placebo and then propranolol 80 mg per day. Although the patients were blinded to the study medication, the investigator knew the identity of the agent. The number of migraine attacks per month diminished from 6.35 during prochlorperazine treatment to 6.25 during placebo treatment and to 3.15 during propranolol treatment.

Successful prolonged use of propranolol for at least one year was reported by Rosen (26). In his open study of 1,036 patients, 865 had been treated with propranolol and 171 were used as a control group that received other migraine treatments. Rosen noted an 84% response rate for the propranolol-treated patients versus a 32% response rate for the control group. In addition, the number of patients who were migraine-free for at least three months during propranolol treatment increased from 390 to 570 after six months of treatment and to 588 at the end of the first year of the study.

In the past several years, a long-acting preparation of propranolol has become available. Diamond and his colleagues (27) recently examined its use in the treatment of headache. Of the 202 patients enrolled in the study, 100 had pure migraine, 6 had pure muscle-contraction headache, and 96 experienced the mixed-headache syndrome; that is, intermittent migraine superimposed on a daily muscle-contraction headache. An excellent response was noted by 24 patients, and another 45 experienced at least a 50% reduction in headache frequency. Only 26 patients reported no improvement in their headaches. Many of these patients reported prior histories of poor response to treatment, so that other medications were used during propranolol therapy. However, of the 80 patients given only long-acting propranolol, 64% achieved at least a 50% reduction in their headaches, and only 9% were treatment failures.

Timolol

Recently, in an open study by Gallagher (28), timolol has been appraised by examination of the dosages of timolol and efficacy in migraine. The six-month study consisted of 116 patients. Of these, 98 completed the entire trial; the remaining patients discontinued the study because of lack of efficacy or adverse effects. Overall headache severity index was reduced from 3.4 to 2.4 by comparing the lead-in to the study to the end of six months of treatment. Fifty-eight of 98 patients achieved at least a 50% reduction in their migraine episodes. An additional 23% of those completing the study reported less than a 25% reduction in their attack frequency. In comparing doses of timolol, the 8 patients on 5 mg daily experienced an average reduction in headache frequency of 65% from a baseline value of 5.4. For the 30 patients on 10 mg per day, a 50% reduction was reported, with 4.2 attacks per month. Similar decreases in headache frequency of about 42% from baseline occurred in 73 patients treated with dosages of up to 30 mg per day. These patients averaged between 4.3 and 4.6 migraines per month. The authors suggest that individual differences in sympathetic tone could result in the dose-variant responses in migraine frequency.

Nadolol

Medina (29) has recently assessed nadolol in an open trial composed of three groups of patients. The first group consisted of patients with pure migraine who had previously demonstrated a partial response to propranolol. The second group was diagnosed as mixed headaches, with a previous partial response to antidepressants. In the third group, the migraine patients had not been treated previously. The first group of patients was merely switched to nadolol for continued prophylaxis. Nineteen patients had a further reduction in their headaches with nadolol. However, 3 reported no further improvement, and 7 experienced an increase in their headaches. In the second group, treated with antidepressants, the addition of nadolol to the treatment regimen resulted in 21 of 46 patients having a further resolution of their headaches. In the third group, previously untreated migraine patients, 75% of 28 patients demonstrated at least a partial response to treatment with nadolol. In comparison to Rosen's study (26), continued improvement in headache frequency was demonstrated with long-term treatment with beta blockers.

Double-Blind Placebo-Controlled Studies
Nonselective Beta-Adrenergic Blockers

Propranolol

In 1972, Weber and Reinmuth (30) reported the first double-blind, placebo-controlled, crossover study of a beta-adrenergic-blocking agent in migraine prophylaxis. They examined the efficacy of 80 mg per day, in divided doses, of propranolol versus placebo in 19 patients who had completed a six-month trial. Four of the 19 patients essentially had a complete remission of migraine during the propranolol portion of the study. An additional 8 had at least a 50% reduction in their migraine frequency or severity. Of these 12 patients, 3 reported a partial response with placebo as well as with the active medication.

Subsequently, Borgesen (31) in a study of 30 patients using 120 mg per day of propranolol, in divided doses, versus placebo, reported a possible response of the patient's migraine to this medication. The single-blind, crossover study, conducted over six months, showed that 9 patients had at least a 50% reduction in their migraines, and another 9 demonstrated at least a partial response.

In a double-blind, crossover study, Diamond and Medina (32) reported on 62 patients who completed the study. The protocol required patients to be randomly given doses of either propranolol 80 mg daily or placebo for a four-week period. The patients then were crossed over to the other study drug. At each succeeding four-week interval, patients could elect to continue treatment or cross over. Every two weeks, the patients also could elect to double the dosage of the treatment drug, if indicated to alleviate the headaches. Of the 62 patients completing the trial, 50 patients used propranolol for eight weeks, 6 patients for six weeks, and 6 patients for four weeks. Thirty-four patients completing the study preferred propranolol over placebo, and 17 considered the placebo more effective. To corroborate the patient's preference, the headache index ratio and relief medication index were evaluated in 27 of the 34 propranolol responders and 10 of the 17 placebo responders. The authors also noted a carry-over response in those patients initially using propranolol who had switched to placebo therapy.

A study undertaken at the University of Granada in Spain (33) involved a small group of nine patients treated with 160 mg per day of propranolol. This crossover study demonstrated a potential effect of reduction of migraine frequency and also demonstrated that propranolol reduced the severity of the attacks.

A double-blind, crossover study was conducted by Stensrud and Sjaastad (34) to evaluate the efficacy of the dextro form of propranolol. Dextro propranolol has no beta-adrenergic-blocking effects. Twenty patients were treated for four weeks, with one-week washout periods between treatment intervals of racemic propranolol, which is the dextroisomer of propranolol, and placebo. The two forms of treatment were given at dosages of 40 mg, four times per day. Treatment with propranolol, both the racemic and dextroisomer forms, demonstrated statistically significant, improved results as compared to placebo. The racemic form demonstrated better results than did the dextroisomer form, although the data were not statistically significant. The authors agreed on the importance of beta-adrenergic-blocking properties, although other pharmacologic properties of the beta blockers may be responsible for the antimigraine effect.

Similar results were found in a study by Hardorfer-Brunc (35) in 44 migraine patients, a portion of whom had concomitant medical conditions for which propranolol was being used. The authors reported that 55.2% of 29 patients who completed the double-blind trial had positive benefits from propranolol. These data were compared to the 27.8% response rate among patients who received placebo.

Long-term benefits of propranolol therapy have been maintained after discontinuation of prophylactic treatment in a multicenter study (36). In the single-blind study, 245 patients were initially treated with placebo for one month and then switched to propranolol therapy for one month. After receiving active drug for one month, 148 patients reported positive effects on their migraine attacks.

These patients were subsequently enrolled in a double-blind, placebo-controlled study. In the second phase of the study, patients were treated for four weeks with either propranolol or placebo. The patients then were given the option of continuing treatment or switching to the alternative study drug. Of the 148 patients entering the second phase, 100 completed the study. In the study, 80 patients were either started on propranolol therapy or, at the end of the first month of phase II, elected to switch to propranolol in a blinded fashion. Patients were allowed to continue therapy for 6 to 12 months. Of those continuing on propranolol for at least 6 months, 75 were subsequently evaluated during an additional 2 month period. During this phase, crossover to the placebo was conducted in a blind manner. A 2 month remission of the migraine attacks during placebo treatment was reported by 35 patients, thus suggesting long-term beneficial outcome from propranolol therapy extending beyond the treatment period. Eight of the 75 patients, however, did experience an increase in the frequency or severity of their migraine, as compared to the period before enrollment in the study.

The majority of propranolol studies in migraine have used dosages of 160 mg per day or less. A recent study (37) by Nadelman and associates examined the effects in migraine of propranolol dosages up to 320 mg per day. This placebo-controlled study continued for 34 weeks. Propranolol was administered in incremental dosages starting with 20 mg four times daily. The dosage was increased every two weeks if the patient experienced any migraine attacks during the study period. Of 62 participants, 33 were progressively advanced to 80 mg of propranolol four times daily. A reduction in headache unit index was reported by 77%, and 84% decreased the types and amounts of abortive medications. A progressive decrease in these indices was seen with continued treatment, and the authors suggested that for those patients with an incomplete response to lower dosages of propranolol, higher dosages of the drug may exert further beneficial effects.

Nadolol

Two studies using placebo control have examined the efficacy of nadolol in migraine. In a study conducted by Ryan and his colleagues (38) in 80 patients with migraine, an initial 8-week phase of placebo treatment was followed by a double-blind enrollment into four treatment groups. The subjects were divided into treatment groups as nadolol 80 mg daily, nadolol 160 mg daily, nadolol 240 mg daily, and placebo. The second phase of the study continued for 12 weeks. At each 4-week interval, headache frequency and severity were averaged for the patients. Considerable variation in headache frequency was demonstrated during the first month of treatment. The frequency ranged from 7.1 headaches per month for those eventually treated with 160 mg per day of nadolol to 8.15 attacks for those who were placed in the placebo group. The data evaluated from the severity index were less variable. However, this index decreased from 15.65 for those who continued on placebo to 15.2 for those who subsequently received 160 mg of nadolol daily. Patients receiving maximal dosage of active medication reported 16.7 on the severity index during the placebo lead-in phase. At the conclusion of the study, all groups had demonstrated at least a 45% decrease in headache frequency (placebo group) to a 71% decrease for those patients receiving 160 mg daily. Similar results were noted in headache severity in all four treatment groups. Statistical analysis was not provided in the report, thus preventing evaluation of the significance of these intergroup comparisons.

In 1984, Freitag and Diamond (39) reported the results of a double-blind study with nadolol, which was conducted similarly to the study by Ryan and his group. Of 32 patients who entered and completed the study, 24 were treated with nadolol and 8 with placebo. In evaluating the outcome, the indices of pain, frequency, intensity, and relief medications were used. No placebo responders were demonstrated in any of the four indices. Thirty percent of the evaluated nadolol cases experienced at least a 50% reduction of the pain index, and 27% had similar reductions in the frequency index, 32% in the intensity index, and 43% at least a 50% reduction in the use of abortive or rescue medications. Although statistically significant differences were not found between varying doses of nadolol, the study outcome yielded significant variations in nadolol-treated patients versus placebo. In addition, 70 of 88 patients treated in an open trial of nadolol for periods of up to two years experienced at least a 50% reduction in migraine attacks.

Timolol

Double-blind studies on the prophylactic use of timolol in migraine have been undertaken. Briggs and Millac (40) conducted a double-blind, crossover trial in 14 patients treated in four study intervals of six weeks. The two groups were randomly selected for treatment with either timolol 10 mg twice daily or placebo. After six weeks, the patients were crossed over to the alternate study drug for another six-week period. The patients then were randomly selected for treatment according to protocol. Statistically significant differences were demonstrated in the second phase of the study for those patients treated with timolol.

Stellar and his colleagues (41) reported on a crossover study of 107 patients treated with timolol in doses of either 20 or 30 mg daily. The study extended over 20 weeks and consisted of an initial 4-week placebo phase followed by 8 weeks of treatment with either placebo or timolol. At the end of the second phase, patients were crossed over to the other treatment group. In the 94 patients completing the study, headache frequency was decreased from the initial phase, with a mean of 6.8 attacks per month, to 4.3 attacks per month in patients on active therapy and 5 attacks per month in the placebo-treated group. No significant variation was demonstrated in this study in comparing the order in which the patient received active medication. The authors also noted that timolol exerted little effect on reducing the mean headache severity or duration of the acute headache attack. At least a 50%

reduction in the frequency of the headaches was reported by 65% of the patients completing the study.

Selective Beta-Adrenergic Blockers

Metoprolol

The beta-1 selective agent, metoprolol, was evaluated in a multicenter Danish study (43). The study consisted of a four-week placebo treatment period, followed by random selection of patients to an eight-week treatment period with either placebo or metoprolol 200 mg daily. Statistical analysis of the two treatment groups failed to demonstrate any difference between the groups at the end of the initial phase in the indices of headache frequency and duration of headaches, severity scores, or the number of abortive medications and doses consumed. During the controlled phase, minimal beneficial changes were noted for those patients continued on placebo. The patients receiving metoprolol demonstrated statistically significant decreases in all parameters. The number of attacks decreased from 4.41 during placebo treatment to 3.11 at the end of the study. Patients treated with metoprolol also reported a decrease in severity and duration of the migraine attacks as compared to placebo. The study was completed by 62 patients.

A study comparing metoprolol and placebo in the prophylaxis of migraine or mixed headaches was conducted at Princess Margaret Migraine Clinic by Steiner and his associates (44). Of the 88 patients who initially received placebo during the first month of the study, 29 placebo responders were eliminated from the study. The remaining patients were randomly selected for treatment either with placebo or metoprolol 50 mg twice daily for a two-month period. Patients who demonstrated an inadequate response to treatment then were selected in a blinded fashion for treatment with either metoprolol 50 mg twice daily, if they had been on a placebo, or metoprolol 100 mg twice daily, if they had been receiving active drug. The authors reported statistically significant decreases in all parameters, except the severity scores, for the patients treated with metoprolol as compared to placebo or baseline evaluation periods. Further significant improvements were demonstrated in patients treated with metoprolol 100 mg twice daily as compared to those patients who received 50 mg twice daily during the second phase.

Atenolol

In a study by Forsmann and his colleagues (45), atenolol 100 mg daily was compared to placebo in a double-blind, crossover study. The study consisted of two treatment periods lasting 90 days, which were interspersed by a 14-day washout phase. From the initial group of 24 patients, 20 completed the study. Data were evaluated according to the effects on the integrated headache, which considered the parameters of headache severity, duration, and frequency. Atenolol was found to be superior to placebo in 19 of 20 patients when evaluating the integrated headache and in 15 of 20 patients when assessing headache frequency.

A subsequent multicenter study (46) reported on 63 patients who completed an 8-week baseline period followed by two treatment periods of 12 weeks divided by a 2-week washout phase. As compared to the study by Forsmann et al. (45), there was a reduction of greater than 50% in 33% of the patients in the integrated-headache indices and 50% in the headache-frequency index during active atenolol treatment. These results were significant compared to placebo treatment for both measured indices.

Beta-Adrenergic-Blocking Agents with Partial Agonist Activity

Three studies have been undertaken in migraine prophylaxis with beta-adrenergic-blocking agents that possess intrinsic sympathomimetic activity or partial agonistic activity. Two of those used, alprenolol and oxprenolol, are selective beta blockers. Acebutolol is a beta-1 selective agent.

Alprenolol was compared to placebo in a double-blind, crossover study conducted by Ekbom (47). Of the 33 patients initially enrolled, 28 completed the trial periods. Only 3 of the patients had a greater than 50% reduction in their migraine attacks. In comparison to placebo, 11 patients preferred alprenolol, and 12 preferred placebo.

Subsequently, Ekbom and Zetterman (48) compared oxprenolol to placebo. The results were similarly disappointing. Five of 30 patients had a greater than 50% reduction in their headaches. However, the majority of these patients reported no preference for placebo or oxprenolol, only six chose oxprenolol, and three chose placebo.

Encouraging results were demonstrated in a study by Nanda et al. (49). The authors compared placebo to acebutolol in a double-blind, crossover study that was completed by 33 patients. Parameters of duration and intensity of the headaches were not improved following treatment. However, both treatment groups demonstrated significant reduction in the frequency of attacks when comparing the first study phase to the crossover phase. The baseline values suggested a strong placebo effect during treatment. At completion of the study, 13 patients overall preferred the acebutolol treatment, as compared to 2 patients who preferred placebo. Although the results of the third study suggest a weak effect of acebutolol in migraine prophylaxis, the data from these studies suggest that agents with partial agonistic effects are not beneficial for migraine prophylaxis.

Comparative Studies

A number of comparative studies have been conducted that compare the efficacy of various beta-adrenergic-blocking agents in migraine prophylaxis. Some studies have sought to establish the efficacy of a particular beta blocker, while other investigations have compared newer agents to a standard measure of efficacy; specifically, the beta-adrenergic blocker. Other studies have compared new beta-adrenergic blockers against older, established agents, such as propranolol.

Propranolol Versus Aspirin

Baldate and his colleagues at the University of Bologna (50) have evaluated aspirin as a potential prophylactic agent for migraine and then compared aspirin to a standard of therapy, propranolol.

Eighteen patients started a double-blind, crossover study, extending over two treatment periods lasting three months, respectively, and divided by a two-week washout period; 12 completed the study. The parameters of headache frequency, duration, and severity were evaluated, and a calculated index based on these values was used as the basis of comparison between aspirin and propranolol. Overall, both agents produced comparable degrees of success for the measured parameters. In this study, a change in the headaches was demonstrated during the crossover to the alternate study drug. Minimal improvement in the headaches was noted after switching from propranolol to aspirin. However, in patients switched from aspirin to propranolol during the second treatment phase, almost complete remission of their headaches was reported by 50% of the cases.

Metoprolol Versus Pizotifen

In Europe, pizotifen has become a standard of comparison for many antimigraine drugs. Velming and his colleagues (51) compared metoprolol in dosages of 50 mg twice daily to pizotifen 0.5 mg three times daily, in a double-blind, crossover study. This study included a four-week washout period between study medications. The frequency and severity of headaches and consumption of abortive medications were used as comparative indices. Although both agents produced significant decreased in headache frequency and severity as compared to the initial phase, neither drug was statistically superior to the other in prophylaxis. The patients treated with metoprolol did not have a significant decrease in the amount of ergot preparations used abortively for migraine attacks as compared to the initial phase. However, these patients encountered less adverse effects during the metoprolol phase as compared to the pizotifen phase. The study was completed by 31 patients.

Propranolol Versus Amitriptyline

Ziegler and his group (52) compared propranolol and amitriptyline, both agents that have been well established as to the clinical and research benefits in migraine prophylaxis. In comparing relative efficacy in migraine, both agents were evaluated for correlating improvement in headaches with improvement in anxiety and depression. This extensive study, which lasted for 40 weeks, involved crossover to the alternative agent. Treatment phases were divided by a washout interval. Thirty of 54 patients completed the study, and 12 reported at least a 50% reduction in headaches following propranolol treatment. Ten patients treated with amitriptyline had similar results. Good response to each agent was reported in 7 patients. Minimal correlations were reported between headache improvement in these patients and the scores on the Zung and Hamilton tests, and on the Spielberger STAI (State-Trait Anxiety Inventory).

Pindolol Versus Clonidine Versus Carbamazepine

In an open trial, Anthony et al. (53) enrolled 153 patients who were assigned to receive one of three medications used in the study. Patients failing to respond to inital therapy, despite an increase in dosage, could be switched to one of the alternative agents. The report did not indicate if the patients were aware of which agents they were using during any of the treatment phases. The authors reported that 41 of 79 patients (52%) had at least a 50% reduction in the frequency of their migraine attacks during therapy with pindolol, a beta-adrenergic-blocking agent with partial agonist activity. Clonidine was administered to 73 patients, and 29 (40%) experienced a similar reduction in the migraine episodes. The data on carbamazepine indicated at least a 50% reduction of headaches in 51 patients (29%) administered this medication.

Beta Blockers Versus Clonidine

Two studies have compared clonidine to beta blockers previously established for migraine prophylaxis. Kass and Nestvald (54) compared clonidine to propranolol in a double-blind, crossover study. This study was completed by 21 patients who received either clonidine 100 mcg daily or propranolol 160 mg daily. At least a 50% reduction in headache frequency was reported by 62% of the patients on propranolol. In comparison, 38% of the patients treated with clonidine had similar results. During propranolol therapy, the use of salicylates for the treatment of headache occurred slightly more frequently than during clonidine-treated periods. However, the use of ergotamine and other analgesics was less during propranolol treatment periods. A decrease in the number of missed workdays due to migraine was reported during therapy. The authors state that the differences were not statistically significant between the two treatment periods.

In a crossover trial conducted by Louis et al. (55), metoprolol and clonidine were compared. The study extended over 24 weeks, and the beta blocker was demonstrated to be more beneficial. For the 23 patients completing this study, clonidine produced no significant differences from the baseline period in the following parameters: frequency, duration, and severity of the attacks, and the number of doses of abortive agents. Metoprolol, however, produced statistically significant difference in all four parameters, as compared to the baseline and clonidine treatment periods.

Although these two studies differ in their assessment of clonidine's efficacy in migraine prophylaxis, both demonstrate the effectiveness of propranolol and metoprolol. Both studies also suggest that beta blockers are more efficacious than is clonidine in migraine treatment.

Beta Blockers Versus Serotonin-Uptake Inhibitors

In two separate double-blind, crossover studies, femoxitine, a serotonin-uptake inhibitor, was compared to propranolol. Each study lasted for six months. Anderson and Petersen (56) reported that in the 37 patients completing the trial, no significant difference was demonstrated between the two treatment periods as to the number of migraine attacks or the number of days with headache. However, propranolol, in contrast to femoxitine, produced a significant reduction in the headache indices of severity and duration.

In the later study by Kangaghiemi et al. (57), 24 out of 29 patients completed the study. Femoxitine failed to produce statistically significant results as compared to the baseline period.

In contrast, the propranolol treatment periods demonstrated significant reductions in all headache parameters. Both of these studies confirmed the benefits of propranolol, but failed to demonstrate the benefits of an experimental serotonin-uptake inhibitor in migraine prophylaxis.

Another serotonin-uptake inhibitor, clomipramine, also has been investigated for migraine prophylaxis. Langohr and his associates (58) compared clomipramine with metoprolol and placebo. The double-blind, crossover study divided 36 patients into five treatment groups. Two groups compared clomipramine and placebo, two groups compared metoprolol and placebo, and the final group compared clomipramine and metoprolol. This particular study demonstrated the significance of statistical methodology in assessing outcome. However, it failed to show that clomipramine was as beneficial as metoprolol in migraine treatment.

Propranolol Versus the Nonsteroidal Anti-Inflammatory Drugs

In 1985, a multicenter study (59) compared naproxyn 110 mg daily, propranolol 120 mg daily, and placebo in a parallel study. In contrast to other studies, the study, involving 129 patients, failed to produce statistically significant differences for either of the active medications over placebo. The parameters that were evaluated included headache frequency and severity. The investigators and patients concurred that naproxyn was superior to placebo. The patients, in contrast to the investigators, considered propranolol better than placebo. Both groups agreed that propranolol was better tolerated than naproxyn.

Another NSAID, tolfenamic acid, was compared to both placebo and propranolol in a double-blind, crossover study by Mikkelsen and his associates (60). Propranolol 120 mg daily was compared to tolfenamic acid 300 mg daily and placebo. The 39 patients were randomly selected for one of the three treatment groups for a 12-week trial, at which time they were crossed over to one of the remaining two groups for another 12 weeks, and finally switched to the remaining treatment for 12 weeks. The study was completed by 31 patients. In evaluating the results, the investigators used the parameters of frequency, severity, and duration of the migraine; the patient's ability to work despite a migraine; and the number of abortive medications used. There was no significant difference demonstrated between propranolol and tolfenamic acid. However, in the treatment period using tolfenamic acid, a slight reduction in the use of abortive therapy was shown.

Johnson and his group (61) compared mefenamic acid 1,500 mg daily, propranolol 240 mg daily, and placebo. Each treatment period lasted three months, and 17 of 29 patients completed the study. During the mefenamic acid treatment period, the number of attacks was slightly reduced. However, this result was not statistically significant as compared to propranolol. Both mefenamic acid and propranolol produced statistically significant results on most parameters as compared to placebo.

Controlled Trials Comparing Various Beta Blockers with Propranolol

Propranolol is currently the standard therapy by which other agents, including other beta-adrenergic-blocking agents, are evaluated for migraine prophylaxis. All currently available beta blockers used in migraine prophylaxis have been compared, in controlled trials, to propranolol.

Atenolol 50 mg twice daily was compared to propranolol 80 mg twice daily in a double-blind, crossover study by Stensrud and Sjaastad (62) Of the 35 patients in the study, 7 reported a high-frequency pattern of headache—up to 34 of 42 days with a headache. After the data of these 7 patients were deleted from further analyses, the results were reviewed and indicated that both propranolol and atenolol significantly reduced the headache indices, including frequency, as compared to placebo. No statistical difference was shown between propranolol and atenolol in their beneficial effect on migraine prophylaxis.

Two studies have compared metoprolol to propranolol. The first study compared metoprolol 100 mg per day to propranolol 80 mg per day (63) in a multicenter setting. Data were collected on 53 pateints, and evaluations were compiled on headache frequency and severity, as well as the use of ergotamine and analgesics. Each treatment received a subjective evaluation. The study consisted of a 4-week placebo washout period between the two active trials. Although both active treatments demonstrated significant results in comparison to placebo, neither produced statistically significant results when compared to each other for any of the measured parameters.

The second study utilized a dose of 200 mg per day of metoprolol versus propranolol 160 mg per day (64). Identical trial methods were used in the second study, except for the doubling of the dosages of both agents. Again, the active treatments produced significant reductions as compared to placebo for all evaluable parameters. However, neither agent was found to produce a better result when metoprolol was compared to propranolol.

Three studies have compared the relative benefits of nadolol against propranolol. Ryan (65) compared two groups of patients treated with nadolol at doses of 80 mg or 160 mg per day to a third group receiving propranolol 160 mg per day. Initially, the patients participated in a placebo-controlled period, and were then randomized into one of the three active treatment groups. Because no statistical comparison was made in this report, it is important to note that during the placebo treatment period, headache frequency averaged from 5.56 attacks per months for those patients receiving nadolol 160 mg per day to as high as 7.42 attacks per months for those patients treated with propranolol. Similar results were found when comparing the headache indices of the 3 actively treated groups as the index ranged from 10.43 for the high-dose nadolol-treatment group, to 14.71 for the propranolol group. This variation causes difficulty for the investigator in proving the assertion that nadolol was the most effective treatment at a dose of 80 mg per day.

The Use of Beta Blockers in Migraine

A subsequent study (66) was conducted that was comprised of 28 patients randomized to receive either nadolol 80 mg per day initially or propranolol 80 mg per day. Following an initial placebo-controlled treatment period of variable length, therapy was started on the two parallel groups. Doses could be adjusted, based on patient tolerance of the active treatments as well as beneficial results on the migraine attacks. Although the two parallel groups demonstrated significant reductions as compared to the placebo phase, no significant differences were demonstrated when the two active treatments were evaluated for their effects on the frequency, duration, and severity of the migraine attacks, or the amount of relief medication utilized.

Lastly, a multicenter trial, placebo-controlled parallel study of nadolol, at either 80 mg daily or 160 mg daily, were compared to propranolol 160 mg daily (67). One-hundred and sixty-eight patients entered into the study and 98 completed and had evaluable data at the conclusion of 12 weeks of active treatment. Twenty-eight patients were excluded during the placebo lead-in phase because of at least a 50% reduction in their headaches during this treatment. Evaluation of the number of headaches, pain and intensity, number of days with headache and relief medications, as well as overall response, found that the lower dose of nadolol and propranolol were statistically equivalent but that at a milligram-equivalent dose, nadolol was more effective than propranolol.

From the Scandinavian Multicenter Headache Trial came a study which compared timolol at 10 mg twice daily to propranolol 80 mg daily in a placebo-controlled double-blind crossover study of the three treatments (68). Data from 80 patients was used in the statistical comparison. Both timolol and propranolol produced significant results compared to baseline for parameters such as frequency of attacks and headache index. Timolol also produced significant results for severity of attacks. Forty-four and forty-eight patients, respectively, had at least a 50% reduction in headache frequency for timolol and propranolol treatment. The two treatments were considered by the researchers to be equivalent to each other in their efficacy in migraine treatment.

Beta-Andrenergic-Blocking Agents Versus Methysergide

Methysergide has also been compared to a beta-1 selective beta blocker, metoprolol and to the nonselective propranolol in an open trial in 134 patients (69). Four treatment groups of patients were utilized in this study. One group was given propranolol starting at 80 mg daily and titrated upwards. This group was made up of patients who had been previously treated with medications for their migraine attacks. The second group received the same treatment but was made up of drug-naive subjects. The last two groups were also drug naive and received either metoprolol at a starting dose of 100 mg daily, which was titrated upwards to 300 mg daily. The last group was given methysergide at doses of 6–10 mg daily based on body size. A total of 93 patients completed the trial. They found that 16 of 25 previously treated patients on propranolol had at least a 50% reduction in the frequency of headaches. This compared to 16 of 24 drug-naive propranolol patients, and 14 of 25 methysergide patients, but only 1 of 16 metoprolol patients. Statistical analysis of those patients, who demonstrated at least some response to their treatment, found that there were significant differences between the two propranolol-treated groups, the drug-naive groups treated with the two beta blockers and between methysergide- and metoprolol-treated patients but not among the other possible treatment comparisons. They concluded that propranolol was an effective treatment and was preferable to methysergide because of reduced problems of adverse experiences.

Multidrug Comparisons

A multicenter trial from Germany compared the efficacy of 5 different agents in migraine prophylaxis (70). The agent used included dihydroergotamine in oral form, to the calcium channel antagonists, flunarizine and nifedipine, to the beta-blocking agents metoprolol and propranolol, during 12 weeks of active treatment after an untreated wash-in period of 8 weeks. The doses utilized were those generally accepted as being effective for migraine prophylaxis based on previous research studies. While statistical analysis comparing each of the treatments was not presented, the results of their study suggested that metoprolol was the most effective therapy followed by dihydroergotamine, propranolol, and flunarizine in that order, with nifedipine showing no efficacy in the prophylactic treatment of migraine.

Prophylactic Therapeutic Trials Summary

From the early case reports, it was evident that the beta-adrenergic blockers had at least some efficacy in the treatment of migraine. Further studies, both in open trials as well as follow-up with controlled studies, demonstrated that not only propranolol but also that other nonselective beta blockers, as well as beta-1 selective blocking agents, lead to significant reduction in the occurrence of migraine attacks.

These open trials lead to placebo-controlled studies of these agents, as well as the newer beta adrenergic blocking agents in attempts to demonstrate their efficacy. Some of these trials also compared the beta blockers to those other therapeutic agents such as amitriptyline and methysergide which had proven track records in migraine treatment. From these studies, it became clear that those beta blockers that lacked partial agonistic effects on the beta receptors were quite efficacious in most controlled trials. Different researchers have utilized different measures of determining outcome prohibiting exacting comparisons of studies. These factors may contribute to some of the differing results noted for each of the beta blockers examined. Statistical analysis and patient selection procedures could also account for some differences noted in different studies. In at least several of the studies, it appears that selection of patients did not necessarily exclude patients with the mixed-headache syndrome, but rather these patients may have been included and asked to evaluate only the migrainous headaches they experienced.

Comparison of the various beta blockers one against the other occurred as it became apparent that propranolol was establishing itself as a gold standard of migraine treatment and the other beta blockers were also being shown to be effective tools for migraine treatment in open and placebo controlled trials. These studies for the most part demonstrated that all those beta-blocking agents without agonistic effects were comparably effective for migraine treatment.

Just as propranolol became the standard by which other beta blockers were evaluated, so newer pharmacologic treatments for migraine such as the nonsteroidal anti-inflammatory agents and the serotonin uptake inhibitors, as well as newer ergot derivatives, and even the calcium channel-blocking agents were compared to the beta blockers. While each of these other classes of agents may have well-defined roles in the treatment of migraine, none of them established themselves to be superior treatments for relief of this disorder.

Special Consideration Therapeutic Trials

Childhood Migraine Prophylaxis with Propranolol

Just as in adults, the problem of frequent and disabling migraine attacks may occur in children and adolescents requiring prophylactic therapy. The usefulness of beta adrenergic-receptor blocking agents have been studied in this group as well.

Ludvingsson reported the first trial of propranolol in children (72). Thirty-two children were enrolled in the study. The doses used were based on body weight. Those under 35 kg received 20 mg three times daily, whereas those over 35 kg were given 120 mg daily. This was a crossover study lasting for 26 weeks with a placebo control. Propranolol treatment reduced the overall frequency of migraine during the study to 3.1 attacks per month compared to the placebo period of 9.3 attacks. The results were statistically significant between the active and placebo treatments. The therapy was well tolerated in general by the patients.

Subsequently, a larger double-blind crossover study was performed in 53 children (72). The dose was begun at 80 mg daily and could be increased if necessary to 120 mg daily. Here, contradictory results were found and no positive benefits from propranolol in any of the evaluable parameters. In fact, they found a statistically significant lengthening of headaches in the propranolol treatment periods.

A trial was also conducted that compared treatment with propranolol to a nondrug therapy, i.e., hypnosis, in 28 patients (73). The children received either propranolol at a dose of 3 mg daily per kg daily, or placebo for 3 months at which time they were crossed over to the alternative therapy for an additional 3 months, at the completion of which they were instructed in self-hypnosis during the last phase of the study. Here, as in the previously cited study, propranolol treatment results were worse than placebo treatment, and self-hypnosis resulted in an approximately two-thirds reduction in headaches.

While these studies present quite contradictory results with regard to propranolol in the treatment of childhood migraine, personal clinical experience suggests that propranolol is an effective treatment for migraine, and may be additionally useful in the treatment of basilar artery migraine (74) and the migraine variant syndrome of abdominal migraine (75).

Propranolol as a Migraine Abortive Agent

After propranolol was becoming established as a migraine prophylactic agent, Tokola and Hokkanen (76) studied its potential use as an alternative to ergotamine for acute migraine treatment. Thirty patients participated in this open trial using in all but one case either 40 or 80 mg of propranolol. Fifty-three percent of the patients had either complete or nearly complete resolution of their migraine attack within 2 hours of administration of the abortive agent. Additionally, 71% of them found propranolol to be as good or better than ergotamine to relieve their migraines based on prior experiences.

Subsequently, Featherstone reported on a series of cases (77) where low doses of propranolol ranging from 10–40 mg would quickly abort migraine attacks. Several of the patients noted that if they combined these low doses of propranolol with aspirin, that this was even more efficacious than propranolol alone.

In a recent double-blind trial at the Diamond Headache Clinic (78), we studied the effects of 10 mg of propranolol alone or with 325 mg of aspirin against placebo. Forty-three patients entered the trial. Only 10 patients, however, responded to this low dose of propranolol, either alone or with aspirin.

Based on the results of these case reports, open and placebo-controlled trials as well as clinical experience with its use, it was found that propranolol may have efficacy as an abortive agent in migraine, but that the dose necessary to achieve relief of migraine acutely is less likely to be at a low dose such as 10 mg, and more likely to be in the range normally used for prophylaxis of migraine of 80–120 mg per attack.

SUMMARY

The role of beta blockers in the treatment of special situations such as pediatric migraine, and as a possible acute-migraine treatment, have been examined. The evidence in pediatric and adolescent migraine is contradictory in the studies that have been conducted. Clinical experience suggests that, while other treatments may be better suited for use in this age group, it appears that propranolol may be a well tolerated alternative treatment in appropriately selected childhood migraineurs.

The same situation also appears to be the case for the use of propranolol for treating acute migraine attacks rather than as a prophylactic agent for this condition, and the trials to date have suggested its efficacy. However, the dose of propranolol that would be potentially effective in the majority of patients remains to be determined in well-controlled trials.

Adverse Experiences of Beta Adrenergic Blockers

While a comprehensive review of beta-adrenergic-blocking agents and their potential for adverse effects is beyond the scope of this present volume, it is worthwhile to consider several adverse-experience problems that have importance in the treatment of the patient with headache.

While a long-term prophylactic benefit has been described above for propranolol, others have described the prompt recurrence of migraine after therapy is discontinued (79). Blank and Reider (80) noted an increased frequency of migraine after beginning treatment with propranolol, the recurrence of migraine

The Use of Beta Blockers in Migraine

attacks after many years of absence (81) or even of the development of classical migraine attacks for the first time in patients without family history of migraine or previous migrainous headaches prior (82).

Over the years, there have been several case reports that have asserted a link between propranolol therapy and the development of migraine complicated by stroke (83-85). However, review of the cases presented by these authors reveals that the patients may have had other risk factors at play in the development of their strokes, such as age (86), previous episodes of hemiplegia unassociated with headache (83), or, as was described by Packard (86), hypertension, obesity, and inadequate treatment of hypertension.

The occurrence of migraine attacks commonly diminishes during the course of pregnancy in most patients. However, for those patients who continued to have migraine during pregnancy, treatment of these attacks is necessary. The use of beta-blocking agents in this situation had not been studied thoroughly however. While their use in the treatment of hypertension and other cardiac-related conditions suggest that they are generally safe (87), there has also been a case reort of fetal demise occurring in a patient who used Inderal as an acute migraine-abortive agent during pregnancy (88). The abstention from drug therapy during pregnancy is the preferred situation so as to avoid any complications in this litiginous age. In those patients with severe, intractable migraine, wherein the patient's general health may be seriously compromised by very frequent migraine attacks, the cautious use of propranolol in a well-informed patient may be a consideration.

Migraine headaches, chronic muscle contraction headaches, and the mixed-headache syndrome, which is characterized by the occurrence of periodic migraine attacks superimposed on a pattern of daily muscle contraction-type headache, have been associated with a depressive etiology (89). The beta-blocking agents have also been associated with the development of depression (90,91). While casual relationships may be difficult to discern in the treatment of patients with migraine and beta blockers, it is important to be aware that these agents, which may benefit the migraine patients, could be involved in the development of an adverse effect such as depression, which may be manifested without the typical mood changes of depression but rather as a masked depression characterized by the evolution of the patient's headaches into the mixed headache syndrome.

Adverse Experience Summary

As with all other pharmacologic agents, the safety of the beta blockers has been examined closely in the vast number of studies undertaken with them. Certainly, they appear to be generally well-tolerated, safe, and efficacious agents in most patients. Appropriate caution, however, is appropriate with these drugs, just as with any other, to minimize the risks of complications that might attend their use.

Several reports have pointed to potential complications of migraine resulting from the use of propranolol. This may certainly also be the situation with the other beta adrenergic blockers used in migraine with their more widespread use.

CONCLUSIONS

The beta-adrenergic blockers have become commonly used to treat a variety of conditions since their introduction into clinical practice. Specific pharmacologic differences lead to one agent having usefulness in a given condition in lieu of a different beta blocker. Here, in the treatment of migraine, these same pharmacologic differences may be seen to account for the beneficial effects of those beta-adrenergic blockers that lack intrinsic sympathomimetic activity or partial agonistic effects being effective in migraine treatment while those that possess this property are not.

Research studies to measure the efficacy of the beta blockers have demonstrated them to be quite comparably effective in head-to-head comparison. Additionally, they are at least as effective as any of the previous or newly developing treatments for the prophylaxis of migraine headache in adult patients. Their use in children and adolescents in controlled studies has raised the question of possible lack of efficacy, yet clinical experience indicates that they certainly may have a strong role to serve in this special situation. Newer methods of utilizing beta blockers are occurring in the other fields of medicine besides headache where they have been examined as abortive agents for migraine, rather than as a preventive agent. Further studies of this application are necessary to assess this use.

Continuing experience with these agents has demonstrated their relative safety and efficacy. While complications or adverse effects do occur with the beta blockers, they do not appear to be any more prevalent than with other agents. These factors all contribute to this group's generally regarded status as the preferential agents for migraine therapy.

REFERENCES

1. Ahlquist, R. P. (1966). The adrenergic receptor, *Pharmaceutical Science, 55(4)*: 359-367.
2. Lands, A. M., Arnold, A., McAnliff, J. P., Ludena L. P., and Brown, T. G. (1967). Differentiation of receptor systems activated by sympathomimetic amines, *Nature, 214*: 597.
3. Middlemiss, D. N., Blakeborough, L., and Leather, S. R. (1977). Direct evidence for an interaction of beta adrenergic blockers with the 5HT receptor, *Nature, 267*: 289-290.
4. Shanks, R. G. (1987). A review of the relationship between beta adrenergic antagonists and their action in migraine, *Advances in Headache Research* (F. C. Rose, ed.), John Libbey, pp. 161-166.
5. Olesen, J. (1986). Beta adrenergic effects on cerebral circulation, *Cephalgia, (suppl. 5)*: 41-46.
6. Edvinsson, L. (1987). Beta adrenoceptor functions and the cerebral circulation, *Advances in Headache Research* (F. C. Rose, ed.), John Libbey, London, pp. 161-166).
7. Fagius J., Sundolf, G., and Wallin, B. G. (1986). Muscle nerve sympathetic activity, with reference to beta adrenoceptor blockade and migraine, *Migraine and Beta Blockade* (J. D. Carroll, V. Pfannenrath, and A. B. Sjaastad, eds.) Hassle, Molndal, pp. 55-61.
8. Schoenen, J. (1987). Sympathetic hyperarousal in migraine? Evaluation by contingent negative variation and psychomotor testing. Effects of

beta blockers, *Advances in Headache Research* (F. C. Rose, ed.), John Libbey, London, pp. 155-160.
9. De Noordhout, A. M., Timsit-Berthier, M., Timsit, M., and Schoenen, J. (1987). Effects of beta blockade in contingent negative variation in migraine, *Ann. Neurol. 21*: 111-112.
10. Joseph R., Steiner, T. J., Schultz, L. U. C., and Rose, F. C. (1985). Does the mode of action of beta receptor blockers in migraine involve alteration of platelet function? *Migraine Clinical and Research Advances* (F. C. Rose, ed.), Kargel, Basel, pp. 115-120.
11. Hedman, C., Winther, K., and Knudsen, J. B. (1986). The difference between nonselective and beta-1 selective beta blockers in their effect on platelet function in migraine patients, *Acta. Neurol. Scand., 74*: 475-478.
12. Kuritzky, A., Ziegler, D. K., Hassanein, R., Sood, P., and Hirwitz, A. (1985). Relation between plasma concentration of propranolol, beta blocking and migraine, *Migraine Clinical and Research Advances Symposium* (F. C. Rose, ed.), Kargel, Basel, pp. 250-255.
13. Cortelli, P., Sacquegna, T., Albani, F., Baldrati, A., D'Alessandro, et al. (1985). Propranolol plasma levels and relief of migraine, *Arch. Neurol. 42*: 46-48.
14. Gengo, F. M., Fagan, S. C., Kinkel, W. R., and McHugh, W. B. (1984). Serum concentrations of propranolol and migraine prophylaxis, *Arch. Neurol., 41*: 1307.
15. Hiatt, W. R., Wolfel, E. E., Stoll, S., Nies, A. S., Zerbe, G. O. et al. (1985). Beta-2 adrenergic blockade evaluated with epinephrine after placebo, atenolol, and nadolol, *Clin. Pharmacol. Ther., 37(1)*: 2-6.
16. V. Slotnick, personal communication.
17. Patel, L. and Turner, P. (1981). Central actions of beta adrenoreceptor blocking drugs in man, *Med. Res. Rev., 1(4)*: 387-410.
18. Jay, G. W., Renelli, D., and Mead, T. (1984). The effects of propranolol and amitriptyline on vascular and EMG biofeedback training, *Headache, 24(2)*: 59-69.
19. Wykes, P. (1968). The treatment of angina pectoris with coexistent migraine, *Practitioner, 200(199)*: 702-704.
20. Bekes, M., Matos, L., Rausch, J., and Torok, E. (1968). Treatment of migraine with propranolol, *Lancet, 2(575)*: 980.

21. Hall, G. H. (1968). Treatment of migraine with propranolol, *Lancet, 2* (*578*): 1139.
22. Sales, F., and Bada, J. L. (1975). Practolol and migraine, *Lancet, 1*: 742.
23. Ljung, O. (1980). Treatment of migraine with metoprolol, *NEJM, 303 (3)*: 156-157.
24. Wideroe, T. E. and Vigander, T. (1974). Propranolol in the treatment of migraine, *Br. Med. J. 2*: 699-701.
25. Nair, K. G. (1975). A pilot study of the value of propranolol in migraine, *Postgraduate Medicine, 21(3)*: 111-113.
26. Rosen, J. A. (1983). Observations on the efficacy of propranolol for the prophylaxis of migraine, *Ann. Neurol., 13*: 92-93.
27. Diamond, S., Solomon, G. D., Freitag, F. G., and Mehta, N. D. (1987). Long-acting propranolol in the prophylaxis of migraine, *Headache, 27 (2)*: 70-72.
28. Gallagher, R. M., Stagliano, R. A., and Sporazza, C. (1987). Timolol maleate, a beta blocker in the treatment of common migraine headache, *Headache, 27*: 84-86.
29. Medina, J. L. (1988). Effectiveness of nadolol in a clinic population of migrainous patients, *Headache, 28(2)*: 99-102.
30. Weber, R. B. and Reinmuth, O. M. (1972). The treatment of migraine with propranolol, *Neurology, 22(4)*: 366-369.
31. Borgesen, S. E., Nielsen, J. L, and Moller, C. E. Prophylactic treatment of migraine with propranolol, *Acta. Neurol. Scand., 50(5)*: 651-656.
32. Diamond, S. and Medina, J. L. (1976). Double-blind study of propranolol for migraine prophylaxis, *Headache, 16(1)*: 24-27.
33. Pita, E., Higueras, A., and Bolanos, J. (1976). Propranolol and migraine. A clinical trial, *Arch. Pharmacol. Toxicol., 3(3)*: 273-278.
34. Stensrud, P. and Sjaastad, O. (1976). Short term clinical trial of propranolol in racemic form (Inderal®), D-propranolol, and placebo, *Acta Neurol. Scand., 53(3)*: 229-232.
35. Hardorfer-Brune, E. and Kaiser, K. (1976). Propranolol in der migraine therapie, *Medizinishe Welt, 28(47)*: 1931-1935.
36. Diamond, S., Kudrow, L., Stevens, J., and Shapiro, D. B. Long-term study of propranolol in the treatment of migraine, *Headache, 22(6)*: 268-271.

37. Nadelmann, J. W., Stevens, M. P., and Spaer, J. R. (1986). Propranolol in the prophylaxis of migraine, *Headache, 26*(*4*): 175-182.
38. Ryan, R. E. and Sudilovsky, A. (1983). Nadolol: Its use in the prophylactic treatment of migraine, *Headache, 23*: 26-31.
39. Freitag, F. G. and Diamond, S. Nadolol and placebo comparison study in the prophylactic treatment of migraine, *JAOA, 84*(*4*): 737-741.
40. Briggs, R. S. and Millac, P. A. Timolol in migraine prophylaxis, *Headache, 19*(*7*): 379-381.
41. Stellar, S., Ahrens, S. P., Meibohm, A. R., and Reines, S. A. (1984). Migraine prevention with timolol, a double-blind crossover study, *JAMA, 252*(*18*): 2576-2580.
43. Andersson, P. G., Dahl, S., Hansen, J. H., Hansen, P. E., Hedman, C., et al., Prophylactic treatment of classical and nonclassical migraine with metoprolol, a comparison with placebo, *Cephalgia, 3*: 207-212.
44. Steiner, T. J., Joseph, R., Hedman, J. C., and Rose, F. C. (1988). Metoprolol in the prophylaxis of migraine: Parallel groups comparison with placebo and dose ranging follow-up, *Headache, 28*(*1*): 15-23.
45. Forssman, B., Lindblad, C. J., and Zbornikova, V. (1983). Atenolol for migraine prophylaxis, *Headache, 23*(*4*): 188-190.
46. Johansson, V., Nilsson, L. R., Widelius, T., Javerfalk, T., Hellman, P., et al. (1987). Atenolol in migraine prophylaxis, a double-blind crossover multicentre study, *Headache, 27*(*7*): 372-374.
47. Ekbom, K. (1975). Aprenolol for migraine prophylaxis, *Headache, 15* (*2*): 129-132.
48. Ekbom, K. and Zetterman, M. (1977). Oxprenolol in the treatment of migraine, *Acta Neurol. Scand., 56*(*2*): 181-184.
49. Nanda, R. N., Johnson, R. H., Gray, J., Keogh, H. J., and Melville, I. D. (1978). A double-blind trial of acebutolol for migraine prophylaxis, *Headache, 18*(*1*): 20-22.
50. Baldrati, A., Cortelli, P., and Procaccianti, G. (1983). Propranolol and acetylsalicylic acid in migraine prophylaxis, *Acta Neurol. Scand., 67*(*3*): 181-186.
51. Vilming, S., Standnes, B., and Hedman C. (1985). Metoprolol and pizotifen in the prophylactic treatment of classical and common migraine, a double-blind investigation, *Cephalgia, 5*: 17-23.
52. Ziegler, D. K., Hurwitz, A., Hassanein, R. S., Kodanaz, H. A., Preskorn, S. H., et al. (1987). Migraine prophylaxis. A comparison of propranolol and amitriptyline, *Arch. Neurol. 44*: 486-489.

53. Anthony, M., Lance, J. W., and Somerville, B. (1972). A comparative trial of pindolol, clonodine, and carbamazepine in the interval therapy of migraine, *Med. J. Aust.*, *1(26)*: 1343-1346.
54. Kass, B. and Nestvold, K. (1980). Propranolol (Inderal®) and clonidine (catapres) in the prophylactic treatment of migraine, a comparative trial, *Acta Neurol. Scand.*, *61(6)*: 351-356.
55. Louis, P., Schoenen, J., and Hedman, C. (1985). Metoprolol versus clonidine in the prophylactic treatment of migraine, *Cephalgia*, *5*: 159-165.
56. Andersson, P. G. and Petersen, E. N. (1981). Propranolol and femoxitine, a 5-HT uptake inhibitor in migraine prophylaxis, *Acta Neurol. Scand.*, *64(4)*: 280-288.
57. Kangagniemi, P. J., Nyrke, T., Lang, A. H., and Petersen, E. (1983). Femoxetine, a new 5-HT uptake inhibitor and propranolol in the prophylactic treatment of migraine, *Acta Neurol. Scand.*, *68(4)*: 262-267.
58. Langohr, H. D., Gerber, W. D., Koletzki, E., Mayer, K., and Schroth, G. (1985). Clomipramine and metoprolol in migraine prophylaxis—a double-blind crossover study, *Headache*, *25(2)*: 107-112.
59. Sargent, J., Solbach, P., Damasio, H., Baumel, B., Corbett, J., et al. (1985). A comparison of naproxyn sodium to propranolol hydrochloride and a placebo control for the prophylaxis of migraine headache, *Headache*, *25(6)*: 320-324.
60. Mikkelsen, B., Pedersen, K. K., and Christiansen, L. V. (1986). Prophylactic treatment of migraine with tolfanamic acid, propranolol, and placebo, *Acta Neurol. Scand.*, *73(4)*: 423-427.
61. Johnson, R. H., Hornabrook, R. W., and Lambie, D. G. (1986). Comparison of mefanamic acid and propranolol with placebo in migraine prophylaxis, *Acta Neurol. Scand.*, *73(5)*: 490-492.
62. Stensrud, P. and Sjaastad, O. (1980). Comparative trial of tenormin (atenolol) and Inderal® (propranolol) in migraine, *Headache*, *20*: 204-207.
63. Olesen, J. E., Behring, H. C., Forssman, B., Hedman, C., and Hedman, G., et al. Metoprolol and propranolol in migraine prophylaxis: a double blind multicentre study, *Acta Neurol. Scand.*, *70*: 160-168 (1984).
64. Kangasniemi, P. and Hedman, C., Metoprolol and propranolol in the prophylactic treatment of classical and common migraine, A double blind study, *Cephalgia*, *4*: 91-96 (1984).

65. R. E. Ryan, Comparative study of nadolol and propranolol in prophylactic treatment of migraine, *Am. J. Heart, 108*: 1156-1159 (1984).
66. Olerud, B., Gustavsson, C. L., and Furberg, B. Nadolol and propranolol in migraine management, *Headache, 26(10)*: 490-493 (1986).
67. Sudilovsky, A., Elkind, A. H., Ryan, R. E., Saper, J. R., and Stern M. A., et al, Comparative efficacy of nadolol and propranolol in the management of migraine, *Headache, 27(8)*: 421-426 (1987).
68. Tfelt-Hansen, P., Standnes, B., Kangasneimi, P., Hakkarainen, H., and Olesen, J., Timolol versus propranolol versus placebo in common migraine prophylaxis: a double blind multicentre trial, *Acta Neurol. Scand.,* 69: 1-8 (1984).
69. Steardo L., Bonuso, S., Di Stasio, E., and Marano, E., Selective and nonselective beta blockers: are both effective in prophylaxis of migraine? A clinical trial versus methysergide, *Acta Neruol. (Napoli), 37(3)*: 196-204 (1982).
70. Scholz, E., Gerber, W. D., Diener, H. C., Langohr, H. D., and Reinecke, M., Dihydroergotamine vs. flunarizine vs. nifedipine vs. metoprolol vs. propranolol in migraine prophylaxis: a comparative study based on time series analysis, *Advances in Headache Research*, (F. C. Rose, ed.), John Libby, London, 1987, pp. 139-145.
71. Ludvingsson, J., Propranolol used in the prophylaxis of migraine in children, *Acta Neurol. Scand, 50(1)*: 109-115 (1974).
72. Forsythe, W. I., Gillies, D., and Sills, M. A., Propranolol (inderal) in the treatment of childhood migraine, *Developmental Medicine and Child Neurology, 26(6)*: 737-741 (1984).
73. Olness K., MacDonald J. T., and Oden, D. L., Comparison of self-hypnosis and propranolol in the treatment of juvenile classic migraine, *Pediatrics, 79(4)*: 593-597 (1987).
74. Bahemuka, M., Basilar artery migraine in a child: excellent response to propranolol, *East African Medical Journal, 58(1)*: 75-79 (1981).
75. Symon D. N. K., and Russell, G., Abdominal migraine: a childhood syndrome defined, *Cephalgia, 6(4)*: 223-228 (1986).
76. Tokola R., and E. Hokkanen, Propranolol for acute migraine (Letter), *Br. Med. J., 14(2)*: 6144-1089 (1978).
77. H. J. Featherstone, Low-dose propranolol therapy for aborting migraine, *West. J. Med., 138(3)*: 416-417 (1983).

78. Unpublished data.
79. Klimek, A. and Pozniak-Patewicz, E., Brief Report: the phenomenon of "drug dependency" in the treatment of migraine with propranolol, *Headache, 17(2)*: 75 (1977).
80. Blank N. K. and Rieder M. J., Paradoxical response to propranolol in migraine, *Lancet, December 8, 2*: 1336 (1973).
81. R. H. Robson, Recurrent migraine after propranolol, *Br. Heart J., 39*: 1157-1158 (1977).
82. C. J. Shrape, Propranolol in the treatment of migraine, *Br. Med. J., 3*: 5929-522 (1974).
83. J. L. Prendes, Considerations on the use of propranolol in complicated migraine, *Headache, 20*: 93-95 (1980).
84. G. L. Gilbert, An occurrence of complicated migraine during propranolol therapy, *Headache, 22*: 81-83 (1987).
85. Bardwell, A. and Trott, J. A., Stroke in migraine as a consequence of propranolol, *Headache, 27*: 381-383 (1987).
86. R. C. Packard, Propranolol....not guilty (letter), *Headache, 27(10)*: 587, (1987).
87. P. C. Rubin, Beta blockers in pregnancy, *N. Engl. J. Med., 305(22)*: 1323-1326 (1981).
88. H. J. Featherstone, Fetal demise in a migraine patient on propranolol, *Headache, 23(5)*: 213-214 (1983).
89. S. Diamond, Depression and headache, *Headache, 23*: 122-126 (1983).
90. Avorn, J., Everitt, D. E., and Weiss, S., Increased antidepressant use in patients prescribed beta blockers, *JAMA, 255*: 357-360 (1986).
91. Pollack, M. H., Rosenbaum, J. F., and Cassem, N. H. Propranolol and depression revisited, three cases and a review, *J. Nerv. Ment. Disease, 173(2)*: 118-119 (1985).

5

The Use of Calcium Channel Blockers in Migraine

Glen D. Solomon *Cleveland Clinic Foundation, Cleveland, Ohio*

INTRODUCTION

Since the early 1980s, calcium-channel-blocking (CCB) drugs have been studied and used in the prophylaxis of migraine headaches and related disorders such as cluster headache, vertigo, and seizures. The CCBs were originally studied because of their ability to inhibit arterial vasospasm and block platelet serotonin release and aggregation (1). However, the effects of CCBs on cerebral blood flow, neurotransmission, and neuroreceptor blockade (2) provide additional mechanisms for their efficacy in migraine prophylaxis.

THE ROLE OF CALCIUM IN VASCULAR SMOOTH MUSCLE

To appreciate the pharmacologic effects of CCBs, the physician must be aware of the role played by calcium in the contraction of vascular smooth muscle. The contraction of vascular smooth muscle is an energy-consuming process, in which myosin both attaches and detaches from the actin filament. When intracellular Ca^{2+} in the smooth muscle increases to approximately 10^{-6} M, Ca^{2+} binds to the calcium-binding protein, calmodulin. The Ca^{2+}-calmodulin complex activates the enzyme myosin kinases; this phosphorylates a light chain of myosin, which permits myosin to interact with actin. The actin-myosin interaction produces contraction of the muscle cell, and, in turn, arteriolar constriction (3).

Knowledge is limited concerning the actual structure of the calcium channels in the cell membrane. However, the channels may be considered as aqueous gates, specifically selective for calcium ions and controlled by voltage (potential) sensors that determine whether the gate is open or closed. Because the movement of Ca^{2+} through these channels is controlled by electrical potentials, they are called *potential-dependent* (or *voltage-operated*) channels (3).

Vascular smooth-muscle contraction can be initiated by the activation of potential-dependent calcium channels and also by the activation of receptor-operated channels by norepinephrine. The entry of Ca^{2+} ions through receptor-operated channels triggers the release of Ca^{2+} from storage sites in the sarcoplasmic reticulum. When the Ca^{2+} concentration increases to appropriate levels, the Ca^{2+}-calmodulin complex is activated and produces smooth-muscle contraction (4).

Although the mechanism of vasoconstriction in migraine remains unknown, the proposed pathophysiology of variant angina, a vasospastic disorder associated with migraine (5), may provide an explanation for the role of calcium in migraine. Zelis and Flaim (5) propose that vasospasm occurs in individuals who have augmented sarcolemmal calcium stores that can be released by normal amounts of the trigger, calcium, resulting from physiologic activation of receptor-operated channels. Thus, CCBs such as verapamil, diltiazem, and flunarizine may express clinical activity by action on different sites within the cell. Verapamil acts to inhibit calcium influx through receptor-operated channels, thereby blocking the trigger release of sarcolemmal calcium. Through effects on the sodium-potassium pump and energy-dependent calcium extrusion, diltiazem decreases intracellular calcium concentrations. Flunarizine is believed to function intracellularly as an inhibitor of intracellular calcium overload.

PHARMACOLOGY OF CALCIUM CHANNEL BLOCKERS

Unlike the beta blockers, the CCBs consist of chemically unrelated compounds. At least five classes of CCBs are recognized: (a) dihydropyridines (nifedipine nimodipine), (b) phenylalkylamines (verapamil), (c) benzothiazepines (diltiazem), (d) diphenylalkylamines (prenylamine, lidoflazine) (6), and (e) piperazine derivatives (flunarizine and cinnarizine) (7).

Because these agents have differing chemical structures and actions on the cell, they vary widely in efficacy and side effects. While these drugs work at different sites on the cell, clinical efficacy (or lack of efficacy) with one CCB does not necessarily suggest efficacy (or lack of efficacy) with an unrelated CCB. To better explain the efficacy of the CCBs studied in migraine prophylaxis, each agent will be reviewed individually.

Verapamil

Verapamil, the first compound to be identified with calcium-antagonist properties, was synthesized in the laboratories of Knoll AG in Germany in 1962 (8). Chemically, it is a papaverine-derived calcium-entry blocker. The pharmacology of verapamil has been examined in numerous studies and appears to be unique among the CCBs. The effects of verapamil on cerebral blood flow, arterial dilation, norepinephrine release, dopamine receptors, serotonin release from both brain and platelets, and opiate withdrawal symptoms provide multiple mechanisms for its efficacy in migraine prophylaxis (2).

The Pharmacology of Verapamil

Hayashi and Toda (9) reported that verapamil was effective in attenuating calcium- and potassium-induced contractions in cerebral and peripheral arteries. Cerebral arteries were more susceptible to verapamil's effect than were either coronary or mesenteric arteries. The contractile response to prostaglandin PGF$_2$ alpha also was attenuated by prior treatment with verapamil (10) in a dose-dependent manner. The response in basilar arteries and middle cerebral arteries did not differ significantly. Vascular relaxation was significantly greater in both cerebral arteries than in the coronary or mesenteric arteries. These studies suggest that verapamil inhibits vasoconstriction, whether induced by calcium, potassium, or prostaglandins, and that the effect of verapamil, although nonspecific for cerebral vasculature, is greater in the cerebral arteries than in other arterial beds.

Leblanc and colleagues (11) evaluated the effects of verapamil on vasospasm in the epicerebral circulation. Platelet-rich plasma mixed with ADP was used to induce vasospasm. This study concluded that verapamil can dilate previously constricted arteries and that dilation is associated with increased cerebral blood flow. These findings suggest that platelet-induced vasospasm can be reversed by verapamil.

In addition to its direct effects on the vasculature, verapamil also interacts with the adrenergic nervous system. Feldman et al. (12) found that verapamil and its metabolite, norverapamil, have an affinity for the beta-2 receptors on lymphocytes. With verapamil, the increase in beta-receptor responsiveness was comparable to that seen with the beta blocker propranolol, a drug commonly used in the prophylaxis of migraine. These researchers postulated that, at expected tissue concentrations, verapamil should induce significant beta-2 receptor blockade. Verapamil's affinity for beta receptors was significantly greater than that of the calcium-entry blockers diltiazem and nifedipine.

The adrenergic effects of verapamil are not limited to beta blockade. Verapamil is a relatively potent alpha-2 adrenoreceptor antagonist (13) that can inhibit the contractile responses to alpha-2 adrenoreceptor agonists such as epinephrine. Galzin and Langer (13) postulate that in vascular smooth muscle, alpha-2 adrenoreceptor stimulation is linked to a potential-dependent slow calcium channel and produces an increase in intracellular calcium, thus resulting in vasoconstriction. Verapamil and other calcium-entry blockers can block this scenario. Alpha-2 adrenergic effects also are responsible for alterations in neurotransmitter release within the brain tissue. The release of neurotransmitter is reduced by the stimulation of presynaptic alpha-2 adrenoreceptors, modulating transmitter release in sympathetic neurons. The mechanism by which the alpha-2 adrenoreceptors reduce noradrenergic transmission is inhibition of calcium influx into sympathetic neurons through a potential-dependent slow calcium channel. Verapamil enhances noradrenergic neurotransmission by blocking the alpha-2 adrenoreceptors that modulate transmitter release through a negative feedback mechanism. The overall effect of verapamil's alpha blockade is to increase the release of norepinephrine in the hypothalamus. The CCB diltiazem lacks this effect. Norepinephrine is thought to act within the central nervous system as an inhibitor of nociceptive transmission (14). Thus, verapamil's adrenergic effects may inhibit both vasoconstriction and nociceptive transmission.

Although hypothalamic levels of norepinephrine are increased, plasma norepinephrine levels are reduced during treatment with verapamil (12). This mechanism may explain why verapamil does not cause tachycardia, a reflex which is observed with other vasodilators.

Verapamil also is active on dopaminergic neurons. Like ergot drugs, verapamil competitively inhibits binding to D-2 dopamine receptors (15). It was the most potent D-2 receptor antagonist of the CCBs tested, incuding diltiazem and the dihydropyridines—nifedipine, nicardipine, and nitrendipine. Since dopamine inhibits prolactin secretion by its action on D-2 receptors and verapamil is a D-2 receptor antagonist, it is not surprising that chronic verapamil treatment causes increased prolactin levels (16). Similar to its effect on noradrenergic neurotransmission, verapamil weakly inhibits neurotransmitter release from central dopaminergic neurons (17).

Murakami et al. (18) reported that verapamil decreased serotonin (5-HT) release from brain tissue. Verapamil also inhibits platelet serotonin uptake and release (19). Because serotonin is considered a prime neurotransmitter in pain modulation and may sensitize nociceptors (14), it is possible that some of the migraine prophylactic response of verapamil may be mediated through its effects on serotonin.

Sicuteri (20) has suggested that migraine mimics the opiate-abstinence syndrome and may represent dysfunction of the endogenous opioid pathways. Chronic morphine tretment increased brain calcium levels by almost 100%. During narcotic withdrawal, calcium content rapidly returned to normal. It was proposed that calcium-entry blockers may prevent the opiate-abstinence syndrome through some direct effect on cerebral calcium. Bongianni et al. (21) found that verapamil reduced most signs of morphine abstinence. Verapamil did not displace naloxone from its binding sites, suggesting a different mechanism of action than opioid receptor blockade.

The pharmacokinetics of verapamil in migraine are summarized in Table 1. Based on a dosage of 480 mg/day, plasma levels of 82 to 240 ng/ml can be detected, with CSF levels of 5.2 to 14.8 ng/ml and a CSF-to-plasma ratio of 0.06 (22). Inhibition of cerebral-artery contraction occurs at verapamil concentrations of less than 0.5 ng/ml (9), inhibition of dopamine D-2 receptors occurs at 2.0 ng/ml (15), impairment of norepinephrine storage occurs at 10 ng/ml (23), reduction of dopamine release occurs at 10 to 100 ng/ml (17), and inhibition of lymphocyte beta-2 receptors occurs at a concentration of 32 ng/ml (12).

Because the pathophysiology of migraine remains uncertain, it is difficult to determine why verapamil should be effective in migraine prophylaxis. The pharmacology of verapamil allows for efficacy in migraine prevention, whether migraine is primarily a disorder of vascular reactivity, neuronal transmission, serotonin sensitivity, or the endogenous opioid system.

Clinical Studies with Verapamil

Two double-blind, placebo-controlled studies have been conducted to evaluate the efficacy of verapamil in migraine prophylaxis. Solomon et al. (1) performed a 12-week crossover study in 12 patients, using a dosage of 320 mg/day. They reported an overall

TABLE 1 Pharmacology of Verapamil in Migraine

1. Calcium blockade
   a. Arterial dilation
   b. Increased cerebral blood flow
2. Adrenergic effects
   a. Reduces norepinephrine levels
   b. Blocks B-2 receptors
   c. Alpha-2 adrenoreceptor antagonist
3. Dopaminergic effects
   a. Inhibits binding to D-2 receptors (ergot-like)
   b. Inhibits neurotransmitter release
   c. Increases prolactin levels
4. Serotoninergic effects
   Reduces serotonin release from brain
5. Opiate withdrawal
   Reduces signs of morphine abstinence

reduction in migraine frequency of 43%, with a mean decrease of 49%. Of the 12 patients, 10 (83%) noted improvement, while 8 (67%) noted a 50% or greater reduction in migraine frequency. No major side effects were reported.

Markley et al. (24) performed a double-blind, placebo-controlled, crossover study using verapamil 240 mg/day for eight weeks in 14 patients. Of the 14 patients, 10 (71%) noted improvement in weekly headache scores, with 4 (29%) reporting 50% or greater improvement. The only side effect reported was mild constipation in 6 patients (43%).

To determine if variations in dosage affected clinical efficacy, Solomon et al. (25) undertook a double-blind, placebo-controlled study comparing verapamil 320 mg/day with verapamil 240 mg/day in migraine prophylaxis. With 320 mg/day dosage, the mean monthly migraine frequency was 3.4; with 240 mg/day dosage, the mean monthly migraine frequency was 5.7—thus demonstrating a statistically significant difference ($p < .05$).

The difference between the mean monthly migraine frequency for placebo and the migraine frequency for the second month of active treatment also was calculated for each subject in this study. This figure measures the average reduction in migraine attacks per month, with a larger number number signifying greater improvement. The average reduction in migraine attacks per month was 3.67 with the 320 mg/day dosage, while with the 240 mg/day dosage, the average reduction in migraine attacks per month was 1.04. This difference also was statistically significant ($p < .05$). These results suggest that the effective dosage of verapamil for migraine prophylaxis is 320 mg/day.

To determine whether the benefits noted in controlled, clinical trials could be replicated in the clinical practice of a referral headache center, Solomon et al. (26) reviewed the charts of 133 headache patients refractory to usual therapy and who were treated with verapamil as part of their headache therapy. Of the 133 patients, 26 (20%) were treated with verapamil as their sole drug therapy. The remaining 80% were treated with other prophylactic medications, including NSAIDs, tricyclic antidepressants, MAO inhibitors (MAOIs), lithium, and methysergide. Overall, 45% of these refractory patients had at least a 50% improvement in headache frequency, while only 5% reported a poor result. Of the 26 patients who received verapamil as sole therapy, 46% had at least a 50% improvement in headache frequency, while 8% noted no improvement or an exacerbation. Nine patients out of 133 (7%) discontinued therapy with verapamil. Two patients stopped because of drug ineffectiveness, fatigue, and constipation. Pregnancy and complete headache relief caused two other patients to stop verapamil.

In addition to migraine, verapamil has been found effective in the treatment of acute cluster attacks (27) and in the prophylaxis of episodic (26) and chronic (28) cluster headaches. In the treatment of acute cluster headache with intravenous verapamil, the mechanism of pain relief is attributed to the blockade of pain-inducing neurotransmitters, rather than to vasodilation.

Adverse effects with verapamil have been reported in up to 41% of patients (28) but these generally were mild and temporary.

In all studies of verapamil, the most commonly reported adverse effect is constipation (Table 2).

Jonsdottir et al. (28) evaluated prophylactic trials using the calcium-entry blockers verapamil, nimodipine, and nifedipine. Verapamil was given to 26 patients with common migraine, and 81% reported beneficial results. Twenty-five patients with classic migraine were treated with verapamil, and 72% reported favorable results. In 34 patients with chronic cluster headache, 79% reported benefit from treatment, and 67% of 33 patients with mixed headache reported benefit from the drug. Overall, 71% of 118 headache patients treated with verapamil demonstrated favorable response to the drug. Beneficial results were reported in 62% of patients treated with nimodipine and in 65% of patients treated

TABLE 2 Side Effects During Treatment with Verapamil

	Verapamil	
Diagnosis	Number of patients	Percentage
Constipation or gastrointestinal complaints	26	53
Peripheral vascular complaints; e.g., flushing	11	22
Cardiovascular complaints, postural hypotension, precordial sensations	13	26
Daily dull bilateral headaches*	3	6
Skin rash	2	4
Muscle pain or cramps	1	2
Behavioral changes (fatigue, nervousness)	8	16
Other	3	6

*Different from usual headaches prior to treatment.

with nifedipine. Verapamil was markedly superior to other CCBs in the treatment of chronic cluster headache and the mixed-headache syndrome. In patients with common and classic migraine, the results were equivalent.

Diltiazem

Diltiazem is a benzothiazepine-class CCB that was originally developed in Japan. Research conducted on diltiazem use in migraine has been limited to an abstract by Riopelle and McCans (29) and a letter by Smith and Schwartz (30).

Riopelle and McCans (29) performed an open-label pilot study fo diltiazem 90 mg/day in 15 patients. Migraine frequency decreased by an average of 37% during the first week and decreased by 86% by the fourth week.

Smith and Schwartz (30) studied the effects of diltiazem for eight weeks in nine patients previously refractory to nadolol therapy. Using dosages ranging from 60 to 90 mg four times daily (mean dosage 75 mg four times daily), significant benefit was demonstrated after eight weeks of therapy.

Neither article specifically addressed adverse effects in using diltiazem for migraine prophylaxis. Diltiazem generally is considered to be the best tolerated CCB. The most commonly reported adverse effects include edema, headache, nausea, and rash. These symptoms have been demonstrated in less than 3% of paients. Contraindications to diltiazem therapy include hypotension, sick-sinus syndrome, and second- or third-degree AV block (31).

Nifedipine

Nifedipine was the first dihydropryidine CCB and was originally developed by the Bayer Company in Germany in 1969 (8). Three studies have evaluated the use of nifedipine in migraine.

Kahan et al. (32) performed a double-blind, placebo-controlled, crossover study in eight patients with both migraine and Raynaud's phenomena. Nifedipine, at a dosage of 10 mg three times daily for one month, significantly reduced the frequency and severity of migraine attacks. The researchers reported a 74% reduction in migraine frequency in their study population.

Meyer et al. (33) performed an open-label trial of nifedipine, at a dosage of 20 mg three times daily, in 20 migraine sufferers, and improvement was noted in 75% of the patients. Jonsdottir et al. (28) treated 66 patients with vascular headache with nifedipine for an average of 4.5 months. Some of these patients had participated in the previously mentioned study by Meyer et al. (33). Of the 66 patients, 13 had classic migraine, 17 had common migraine, 19 had chronic cluster, and 17 had mixed headache. Nifedipine was given at dosages between 30 and 120 mg per day, divided into three daily doses. Decreases in the frequency and severity of headache were reported by 65% of the patients. The patients with classic migraine demonstrated the best response, with 77% reporting benefit. Patients with mixed headache showed the poorest response, with 41% reporting benefit. Sixty-five percent of the patients with common migraine reported benefit, and 60% of patients with chronic cluster noted improvement.

In all the studies, adverse effects from nifedipine were commonly reported. In the study by Jonsdottir et al. (28), 71% of the patients noted side effects, as compared with 41% with verapamil and 21% with nimodipine (Table 3). Postural hypotension was the most common symptom, occurring in 53% of the patients. Vascular symptoms such as edema and flushing were observed in 45% of the patients, and gastrointestinal complaints were reported by 28%.

Nimodipine

Nimodipine, like nifedipine, also is a dihydropryidine CCB developed by the Bayer Company in Germany. Nifedipine is believed to differ from nimodipine in that it has a much greater selectivity for cerebral blood vessels than for the peripheral vasculature (34). Nimodipine blocks both receptor-operated channels and potential-sensitive channels (35). Cerebral blood vessels are particularly sensitive to blockade of potential-dependent channels, and less

TABLE 3 Side Effects During Treatment with Nifedipine

Diagnosis	Nifedipine Number of patients	Percentage
Constipation or gastrointestinal complaints	13	28
Peripheral vascular complaints; e.g., flushing	21	45
Cardiovascular complaints, postural hypotension, precordial sensations	25	53
Daily dull bilateral headaches*	4	8
Skin rash	2	4
Muscle pain or cramps	2	4
Behavioral changes (fatigue, nervousness)	6	13
Other	2	4

*Different from usual headaches prior to treatment.

sensitive to stretch-dependent channel blockade. Nimodipine selectively reduces cerebral vascular tone and increases cerebral blood flow (36). Unlike verapamil, nimodipine has no effect on serum norepinephrine levels or cardiovascular reflexes (37). Pharmacokinetically, oral nimodipine is well absorbed, with peak concentrations between one and two hours postdose and a half-life of about three hours (38). In a number of studies, nimodipine has been evaluated for efficacy in vascular headache.

Gelmers (39) performed a double-blind, placebo-controlled, parallel group study in 60 patients, using nimodipine 40 mg three times daily for 13 weeks. From the eighth week on, nimodipine was significantly more effective than placebo. An improvement of 50% or greater was observed in 69% of the patients.

Meyer and Hardenberg (40) studied 27 patients with migraine to compare a nimodipine dosage of 40 mg three times daily with a dosage of 20 mg three times daily. In their double-blind, crossover study of 18 weeks duration (two 8-week treatment periods and a 2-week washout period), headache frequency was significantly reduced at both dosage levels. Improvement began 2 to 4 weeks after initiating therapy. Overall, 78% of patients noted benefit with low dosages of nimodipine, while 93% of patients noted benefit from 40 mg three times daily.

Jonsdottir et al. (28) used nimodipine to treat 85 patients with vascular headaches for an average of 6.5 months. Some of these patients had previously participated in the study by Meyer and Hardenberg (40). Of these 85 patients, 22 had classic migraine, 19 had common migraine, 32 had cluster headache, and 12 had mixed headache. Decreases in the frequency and severity of headache were reported by 62% of the patients. The patients with common migraine demonstrated the best response, with 84% reporting benefit. The patients with mixed headache showed the poorest response, with 33% reporting benefit. In patients with classic migraine, 73% reported benefit, and 53% of patients with cluster headache noted improvement.

Havanka-Kanniainen et al. (41) studied the efficacy of nimodipine (30 mg four times daily) in a 16-week (8 weeks on active drug), placebo-controlled, double-blind, crossover study of 33 patients. They reported an overall reduction in migraine frequency of 28%, while 10 of 33 patients (33%) noted 50% or greater improvement in migraine frequency.

Jensen et al. (42) studied the effect of a single, sublingual 40-mg dose of nimodipine to treat acute classic migraine attakcs. The study was limited due to a high (46%) dropout rate and other methodological difficulties, and nimodipine did not demonstrate beneficial results in migraine-abortive therapy.

Nimodipine was evaluated in the treatment of headache in chronic cerebral ischemia in a double-blind, parallel group study (43) of 65 patients (32 using active drug). Both placebo and active drug were very effective, with no significant differences noted.

DeCarolis and colleagues (44) studied the effect of nimodipine in episodic cluster headache in a pilot study of 13 patients. Using a dosage of 30 mg four times daily, 7 out of 13 patients (53%)

noted cessation of cluster attacks within 10 days. Prior to relief, the average duration of therapy was 5 days. Therapy, when successful, was continued for 30 days before the nimodipine was tapered off and then discontinued.

Side effects reported with nimopidine included muscular pain or cramps and vascular complaints (Table 4). Jonsdottir et al. (28) reported fewer adverse effects with nimodipine than with verapamil or nifedipine. Muscular complaints were more common with nimodipine, but flushing was less common.

In addition to its efficacy in the treatment of vascular headache, nimodipine has been evaluated in the reduction of morbidity in both subarachnoid hemorrhage (45) and stroke (46). In both instances, the drug was proven effective.

TABLE 4 Side Effects During Treatment with Nimodipine

Diagnosis	Nimodipine Number of patients	Percentage
Constipation or gastrointestinal complaints	8	47
Peripheral vascular complaints; e.g., flushing	2	11
Cardiovascular complaints, postural hypotension, precordial sensations	4	22
Daily dull bilateral headaches*	0	0
Skin rash	1	5
Muscle pain or cramps	3	17
Behavioral changes (fatigue, nervousness)	0	0
Other	1	5

*Different from usual headaches prior to treatment.

Flunarizine

Flunarizine is a difluorinated-piperazine-derivative CCB with selectivity for the cerebral vasculature. It was developed by Janssen Pharmaceutica in Belgium and, since 1980, has been studied in the prophylaxis of migraine. Unlike many other CCBs, flunarizine has been the subject of many open trials and over 14 double-blind, controlled studies in migraine prophylaxis (47).

Amery and colleagues (47) compiled the data from seven studies (48-54) performed in Europe in which flunarizine was given at a daily dosage of 10 mg for at least three months. The patient population was 202 subjects between the ages of 13 and 65 (median age was 38). The group included 144 females and 58 males, all with the diagnosis of migraine (classic 54, common 148). A global evaluation was available for 175 patients, and 85.7% of patients reported benefit. Of the group studied, 58.9% reported that the drug was "certainly effective." Flunarizine therapy was marked by progressive improvement over the first three months. After one month of treatment, 61.9% of the patients had a reduction in attack frequency, and after three months, 83.2% of the patients had a reduction in attack frequency. During the third month, 41% of the patients were headache-free. In a long-term study of 125 patients treated for at least one year with flunarizine, the beneficial effects plateaued after three to four months and were maintained thereafter. Analysis of patient characteristics demonstrated that patients with a shorter duration of disease responded better to flunarizine than did patients with a longer history of migraine. Patients younger than 35 had better results than did patients over age 35. The response to flunarizine was not influenced by patient sex, weight, or type of migraine. The only significant adverse effects reported were weight gain, increased appetite, and somnolence.

Only one U.S. study of flunarizine in migraine prophylaxis has been published. However, several studies currently are being conducted. Diamond and Schenbaum (55) studied 20 patients in a single-blind, crossover study comparing flunarizine, 10 mg at bedtime, with placebo. Of the 20 patients, 14 noted an average reduction of 50.5% in headache unit index over the three- to seven-month (12 weeks of active drug) trial. Reported side effects included fatigue or lethargy in 40% of the subjects, and 75% reported weight gain, although it was less than 10% of body weight in all but one patient.

Flunarizine is the only CCB that has been evaluated in the prophylaxis of pediatric migraine. Caers et al. (56) reviewed four studies (57-60) involving 156 children. Most children were treated with a dosage of 5 mg daily. Eight-two percent of the pediatric subjects responded to flunarizine therapy, with 60% of the patients noting a 50% or greater reduction in migraine frequency. Similar to the findings in the studies of the adult population, flunarazine was more effective after three months of therapy than after one month. Adverse reactions in children were seen in 21% of patients, with weight gain and somnolence being the most common.

Sublingual flunarizine has been studied in the acute treatment of the migraine attack. Bonuso et al. (61) studied sublingual flunarizine 10 mg in both isosorbide-dinitrate-induced migraine attacks and in spontaneous migraine attacks and found significant efficacy. When flunarizine was compared with intramuscular ergotamine tartrate 0.25 mg, the flunarizine was found to be equally effective (75% versus 70%). Flunarizine has a latency of drug effect for 14 minutes as compared with 26 minutes for ergotamine. Side effects were not observed with flunarizine use. However, ergotamine triggered nausea, vomiting, fatigue, and chest pressure.

One particular concern with flunarizine is the report of tardive dyskinesia, parkinsonism, and depression in several patients treated with dosages from 5 to 40 mg per day (62,63). Prescribers should exercise caution in treating patients with high doses of flunarizine, and patients should be evaluated for depression and extapyramidal symptoms every three months (63). Tardive dyskinesia has not been reported with other CCBs currently used in migraine prophylaxis.

COMPARISONS OF CALCIUM CHANNEL BLOCKERS

It is apparent from the data previously presented that the five CCBs discussed herein are superior to placebo in preventing migraine attacks. From the clinical viewpoint, it is important to compare these drugs with conventional therapy. Several of these agents have been compared with beta blockers, methysergide, pizotifen, or other CCBs. Virtually all of these studies found no differences between standard therapy and CCBs. However, a large number of subjects are required to differentiate between two effective therapies, a factor lacking in these studies.

Steardo et al. (64) compared flunarizine 10 mg nightly with methysergide 4 mg daily, in 104 patients (53 flunarizine, 51 methysergide) treated for five months. They found that both drugs reduced migraine frequency and duration to a similar extent, whereas flunarizine also reduced migraine intensity. Seven patients discontinued methysergide therapy, five for gastric disturbance and two with peripheral circulatory insufficiency. There were no withdrawals in the flunarizine group, although four patients noted transient drowsiness.

Flunarizine also has been compared with pizotifen, an antiserotonin agent in migraine prophylaxis, in seven European trials (7,47,48,65-68). The studies enrolled 293 patients, 152 on flunarizine and 141 on pizotifen (Table 5). Overall efficacy was similar with both drugs. No individual study found a statistical superiority of flunarizine over pizotifen; however, pooled data do reach statistical significance. Adverse effects were similar with both drugs, with weight gain and somnolence noted by approximately 20% of patients.

Propranolol, a nonselective beta blocker, is considered by many U.S. headache researchers to be the gold standard for migraine prophylaxis. Two CCBs, flunarizine and verapamil, have been compared with propranolol. Soyka and Oestreich (69) studied 434 migraine patients in a parallel group, double-blind study. Good or excellent results were seen in 104 of 166 patients on flunarizine and 105 of 170 patients on propranolol. Side effects were noted by 24.6% of patients on flunarizine and 29.6%

TABLE 5 Global Result in Comparative Trials: Flunarizine Versus Placebo and Versus Pizotifen

	Percentage of patients			
	Reference: placebo		Reference: pizotifen	
Result	Flunarizine (n = 45)	Placebo (n = 46)	Flunarizine (n = 74)	Pizotifen (n = 60)
Excellent	51.1	8.7	59.5	26.7
Good	33.3	41.3	32.4	31.7
Poor	15.6	50.0	8.1	41.6
Intergroup difference*	$p = .001$		$p = .009$	

*Mann-Whitney U test.

of patients treated with propranolol, with the most common symptoms being fatigue, vertigo, and weight gain. A small, double-blind, crossover study of 15 patients compared verapamil 240 mg per day with propranolol, 120 mg per day (70). No signficant differences in efficacy were observed. Constipation was more common with verapamil, whereas fatigue and light-headedness occurred more frequently with propranolol.

Studies comparing the efficacy of CCBs in migraine prophylaxis have been rare. One controlled study and one review of clinical experience with three agents (28) have been published. Bussone et al. (71) studied 25 patients in a 12-week, double-blind, parallel study of flunarizine 10 mg daily versus nimodipine 40 mg three times daily. Both drugs were effective in reducing migraine frequency, but nimodipine had a shorter latency of effect (Table 6). Side effects were less frequent and milder with nimodipine than with flunarizine.

Jonsdottir et al. (28) evaluated prophylactic trials from their laboratory using the CCBs verapamil, nimodipine, and nifedipine (Table 7). They concluded that nifedipine appeared to be more

TABLE 6 Headache Index (HI) Before, During, and After a 12-Week Treatment with Nimodipine or Flunarizine

	Nimodipine (n = 12)	p	Flunarizine (n = 13)	p
Before treatment	258.4 ± 211.3		286.6 ± 352.1	
After 4 weeks	179.1 ± 100.9	<.05 vs. baseline	276.0 ± 326.4	n.s.
After 8 weeks	119.8 ± 68.3	<.001 vs. baseline	202.5 ± 269.1	<.002 vs. baseline <.005 vs. 4 week
After 12 weeks	116.9 ± 105.0	<.001 vs. baseline	200.4 ± 301.8	<.005 vs. 4 week <.002 vs. baseline

*Arithmetic means standard deviation.

TABLE 7 Comparison of Calcium Channel Blockers in Headache

	Percentage reporting benefit		
	Verapamil	Nimodipine	Nifedipine
Classic migraine	72	73	77
Common migraine	81	84	65
Cluster headache	79	53	60
Mixed headache	67	33	41

effective than verapamil or nimodipine in classic migraine, whereas verapamil was most effective in treating mixed headache. They also concluded that verapamil was the drug of choice for treating chronic cluster headache. Of the three drugs studied, nimodipine was the best tolerated, and nifedipine was the least tolerated.

CONCLUSION

The CCBs have revolutionized the management of cardiovascular diseases such as angina pectoris, variant angina, and hypertension and eventually may become the standard therapy for migraine and cluster headaches. A large body of research confirms that these drugs are effective in migraine prophylaxis. The dual questions of long-term safety and benefit compared with other agents have yet to be answered satisfactorily.

Any review of CCBs is incomplete without addressing two topics: when CCBs should be used and which CCB should be selected. Migraine patients who are candidates for CCB therapy include (a) patients refractory to beta-blocker therapy, (b) patients contraindicated to beta blockers (absolute or relative), (c) patients who experienced significant adverse effects or intolerance to beta blockers, and (d) patients with migraine and concomitant medical conditions that are responsive to CCB therapy (i.e., angina pectoris,

TABLE 8 Comparison of Drugs—Efficacy

Drug	Decrease of migraine frequency, %	Patients improved, %	Patients 50% improved, %
Flunarizine	50	87	44
Nimodipine	28	93	48
Verapamil	49	81	46
Nifedipine	74	75	N/A
Diltiazem	64	N/A	N/A

TABLE 9 Comparison of Drugs—Side Effects

Drug	CNS/ behavioral/ sedation	Percentage of patients Muscular	Vascular	Gastric/ constipation
Flunarazine	18	15	0	11
Nimodipine	23	34	6	16
Verapamil	0	0	23	17
Nifedipine	13	0	39	13
Diltiazem	N/A	N/A	N/A	N/A

supraventricular tachyarrhythmias, Raynaud's phenomena) (1). Patients with chronic cluster headache should be cosidered for therapy with verapamil, either as a drug of first choice (28) or as an alternative to lithium therapy. Patients with complicated migraine, hemiplegic migraine, and acephalic migraine (migraine equivalents) also may be excellent candidates for treatment with CCBs.

The best way to select a CCB for migraine treatment would be to review a blinded study comparing the various drugs for efficacy, safety, and adverse effects. Since this type of study has not yet been undertaken, the next best option is to perform a literature search for this data. A review article (72) was last published in 1985, based on English-language articles published before March 1985. This study concluded that there were no major differences among the CCBs with regard to efficacy in migraine (Table 8), but there were differences in the quality and frequency of adverse effects (Table 9). Several additional studies and a comparison trial of nimodipine versus flunarizine (71) have been published since the review article; the conclusions continue to be valid.

REFERENCES

1. Solomon, G. D. and Spaccavento, L. J. (1983). Verapamil prophylaxis of migraine: A double-blind, placebo-controlled trial, *JAMA, 250*: 2500-2502.

2. Solomon, G. D. (1987). Clinical efficacy of verapamil in migraine prophylaxis, *Gynecological Endocrinology, 1* (suppl 3): 28.
3. Braunwald, E. (1982). Mechanism of action of calcium-channel blocking agents, *NEJM, 307*(26): 1618-1627.
4. Zelis, R. and Flaim, S. F. (1982). Calcium influx blockers and vascular smooth muscle: Do we really understand the mechanisms? *Ann. Intern. Med., 94*(1): 124-126.
5. Miller, D., Waters, D. C., Warnica, W., Szlachcic, J., Kreeft, J., and Theroux, P. (1981). Is variant angina the coronary manifestation of a generalized vasospastic disorder? *NEJM, 304*: 763-766.
6. Murphy, K. M. M., Gould, R. J., Largent, B. L., and Snyder, S. H. (1983). A unitary mechanism of calcium antagonist drug action, *Proc. Natl. Acad. Sci. USA, 80*: 860-864.
7. Rascol, A., Montastruc, J. L., and Rascol, O. (1986). Fluanrizine vs. pizotifen: A double-blind study in the prophylaxis of migraine, *Headache, 26*: 83.
8. Flecenstein, A. (1983). History of calcium antagonists, *Circ. Res., 52* (suppl 1): 3-16.
9. Hayashi, S. and Toda, N. (1977). Inhibition of CD2+, verapamil and papaverine, *Br. J. Pharmac., 60*: 35-43.
10. Shimizu, K., Ohta, T., and Toda, N. (1980). Evidence for greater susceptibility of isolated dog cerebral arteries to antagonistis than peripheral arteries, *Stroke, 11*(3): 261.
11. Leblanc, R., Feindel, W., Yamamoto, L., and Milton, J., et al. (1984). The effects of calcium antagonism on the epicerebral circulation in early vasospasm, *Stroke, 15*(6): 1017.
12. Feldman, R., Park, G., and Lai, C. (1985). The interaction of verapamil and norverapamil with B-adrenergic receptors, *Circulation, 72*(3): 547-554.
13. Galzin, A. M. and Langer S. Z. (1983). Presynaptic β_2-adrenoceptor antagonism by verapamil but not by diliatzem in rabbit hypothalamic slices, *Br. J. Pharmac., 78*: 571-577.
14. Field, H. (1987). *Pain*, McGraw-Hill, New York.
15. DeVries, D. and Beart, P. (1985). Competitive inhibition of (^{3}H) Spiperone binding to D-2 dopamine receptors in striatal homogenates by organic calcium channel antagonists and polyvalent cations, *European J. of Pharmac., 106*: 133-139.

16. Maestri, E., Camellini, L., and Rossi, G., et al., (1985). Effects of five days verapamil administration on serum GH and PRL levels, *Horm. Metabol. Res., 17*: 482.
17. Starke, K., Spath, L., and Wichmann, T. (1984). Effects of verapamil, diltiazem and ryosidine on the release of dopamine and acetylcholine in rabbit caudate nucleus slices, *Naunyn-Schmiedeberg's Arch. Pharmacol., 325*: 124-130.
18. Murakami, H., Kaji, E., and Segawa, T. (1978). Influences of verapamil, X-537A, A-23187 and adenosine 3',5'-cyclic monophosphate on release of 5-hydroxytryptamine from rat brain slices, *Japan J. Pharmacol., 28*: 589-596.
19. McGoon, M., Vlietstra, R., and Holmes, D., et al. (1982). The clinical use of verapamil, *Mayo Clin. Proc., 57*: 495-510.
20. Sicuteri, F. (1983). Is acute tolerance to 5-hydroxytryptamine opioid dependent? Its absence in migraine sufferers, *Cephalgia, 3*: 187-190.
21. Bongianni, F., Carla, V., and Moroni, F., et al. (1986). Calcium channel inhibitors suppress the morphine-withdrawal syndrome in rats, *Br. J. Pharmacol., 88*: 561-567.
22. Doran, A., Narang, P., and Meigs, C., et al. (1985). Verapamil concentrations in cerebrospinal fluid after oral administration, *NEJM, 312(19)*: 1261.
23. Zsoter, T., Wolchinsky, C., and Endrenyi, L. (1984). Effects of verapamil on (^{3}H) norepinephrine release, *J. Cardio. Pharmacol. 6*: 1060-1066.
24. Markley, H., Cheronis, J., and Piepho, R. (1984). Verapamil prophylactic therapy of migraine, *Neurology (Cleveland), 34*: 973-976.
25. Solomon, G. D. and Diamond, S. (1987). Verapamil in migraine prophylaxis: Comparison of dosages, *Clin. Pharmacol. Ther., Feb.*: 202.
26. Solomon, G. D., Mehta, N., Freitag, F. G., and Diamond, S. "Verapamil in Refractory Headache Patients," (Abstract) Proceedings of the 3rd Congress of the International Headache Society, Cephalgia.
27. Boiardi, A., Gemma, M., Porta, E., Peccarisi, C., and Bussone, G. (1986). *Ital. J. Neurol. Sci., 7*: 531-534.
28. Jonsdottir, M., Meyers, J. S., and Rogers, R. L. (1987). Efficacy, side effects and tolerance compared during headache treatment with three different calcium blockers, *Headache, 27*: 364-369.

29. Riopelle, R. J. and McCans, J. L. (1982). A pilot study of the calcium antagonist diltiazem in migraine syndrome prophylaxis, *Can. J. Neurol. Sci., 9*: 269.
30. Smith, R. and Schwartz, A. (1984). Diltiazem prophylaxis in refractory migraine, *NEJM, 310*: 1327-1328.
31. *Physician's Desk Reference* (1988). (E. R. Barnhart, ed.), Medical Economics Company, Cradell, New Jersey, pp. 1221-1222.
32. Kahan, A., Weber, A., and Amor, B., et al. (1983). Nifedipine in the treatment of migraine in patients with Raynaud's phenomenon, *NEJM, 308*: 1102-1103.
33. Meyer, J. S., Dowell, R., Mathew, N., et al. (1984). Clinical and hemodynamic effects during treatment of vascular headaches with verapamil, *Headache, 24*: 313-321.
34. Peroutka, S. J., Banghart, S. B., and Allen, G. S. (1984). Relative potency and selectivity of calcium antagonists used in the treatment of migraine, *Headache, 24*: 55-58.
35. Bevan, J. A. and Hwa, J. T. (1985). Calcium channel blockers and vascular tone, *Nimodipine–Pharmacological and Clinical Properties* (E. Betz, K. Deck, and F. Hoffmeister, eds.), F. K. Schattauer Verlag, Stuttgart, New York, pp. 9-17.
36. Kazda, S., Garthoff, B., and Luckhaus, G. (1985). Prevention of acute and chronic cerebrovascular damage with nimodipine in animal experiments, *Nimodipine–Pharmacological and Clinical Properties* (E. Beta, K. Deck, and F. Hoffmeister, eds.), F. K. Schattauer Verlag, Stuttgart, New York, pp. 31-44.
37. Havanka-Knanniainen, H., Juujarvi, K., Tolonen, U., and Myllyla, V. V. (1987). Cardiovascular reflexes and plasma noradrenaline levels in migraine patients before and during nimodipine medication, *Headache, 27*: 39-44.
38. Savage, I. T. and James I. M. (1985). The effect of nimodipine on the cerebral circulation in normal volunteer subjects, *Nimodipine–Pharmacological and Clinical Properties* (E. Beta, K. Deck, and F. Hoffmeister, eds.), F. K. Schattauer Verlag, Stuttgart, New York, pp. 177-184.
39. Gelmers, H. J. (1983). Nimodipine, a new calcium antagonist in the prophylactic treatment of migraine, *Headache, 23*: 106-109.
40. Meyer, J. S. and Hardenberg, J. (1983). Clinical effectiveness of calcium entry blockers in prophylactic treatment of migraine and cluster headaches, *Headache, 23*: 266-277.

41. Havanka-Kannisinen, H., Hokkanen, E., and Myllyla, V. V. (1985). Efficacy of nimodipine in the prophylaxis of migraine, *Cephalgia, 5*: 39-43.
42. Jensen, K., Tfelt-Hansen, P., Lauritzen, M., and Olesen, J. (1985). Clinical trial of nimodipine for single attacks of classic migraine, *Cephalgia,*
43. Hadjiev, D., Velcheva, I., and Ivanova, L. (1985). Nimodipine in the treatment of headache in chronic cerebral ischemia, *Cephalgia, 6*: 131-134.
44. De Carolis, P., Baldrati, A., Agati, R., De Capoa, D., D'Alessandro, R., and Sacquegna, T. (1987). Nimodipine in episodic cluster headache: Results and methodological considerations, *Headache, 27*: 397-399.
45. Allen, G. S., Ahn, H. S., and Preziosi, T. J., et al. (1983). Cerebral arterial spasm' A controlled trial of nimodipine in subarachnoid hemorrhage patients, *NEJM, 308*: 619-624.
46. Gelmers, H. J., et al. (1988). Nimodipine for acute ischemic stroke, *NEJM, 318*: 203-207.
47. Amery, W. K., Caers, L. J., and Aerts, T. J. L. (1985). Flunarizine, a calcium entry blocker in migraine prophylaxis, *Headache, 25*(5): 249-254.
48. Louis, P. and Spierings, E. L. H. (1982). A comparison of flunarizine (Sibelium) and pizotifen (Sandomigran) in the treatment of migraine. A double-blind study, *Cephalgia, 2*: 197-203.
49. Almelo Study Group, Prophylaxis of migraine: comparison of the calcium-entry blocker flunarizine and pizotifen. In preparation.
50. Rascol, A. Double-blind comparison of flunarizine and pizotifen in the prevention of migraine. In preparation.
51. Sorensen, P. S., Hansen, K., and Olesen, J. (1986). Prophylactic effect of flunarizine in patients with common migraine. A double-blind cross-over comparison with placebo, *Cephalgia, 6*: 7-14.
52. Frenken, C. W. G. M. and Nuijten, S. T. M. (1984). Flunarizine, a new preventive approach to migraine. A double-blind comparison with placebo, *Clin. Neurol. Neurosurg., 86*: 17-20.
53. Louis, P. (1981). A double-blind placebo-controlled prophylactic study of flunarizine (Sibelium®) in migraine, *Headache, 21*: 235-239.
54. Ansink, B. J. J., Danby, M., Oosterveld, W. J., and Schimsheimer, R. J. (1983). "The Influence of the Calcium-Entry Blocker Flunarizine on Migraine and on the Vestibular System in Migraine Patients," interim

findings presented at the 12th Scandinavian Migraine Society Meeting, Finland.
55. Diamond, S. and Schenbaum, H. (1983). Flunarizine, a calcium channel blocker, in the prophylactic treatment of migraine, *Headache, 23*: 39-42.
56. Caers, L. I., De Beukelaar, F., and Amery, W. K. (1987). Flunarizine, a calcium-entry blocker, in childhood migraine, epilepsy, and alternating hemiplegia, *Clin. Neuropharmacol., 10*(2): 162-168.
57. Sorge, F. and Marano, E. (1985). Flunarizine vs. placebo in childhood migraine. A double-blind study, *Cephalgia, 5 (suppl. 2)*: 145-148.
58. Sorge, F., De Simone, R., Marano, E., Orefice, G., and Carrieri, P. (1985). Efficacy of flunarizine in the prophylaxis of migraine in children: A double-blind, crossover controlled study, *Cephalgia, 5 (suppl 3)*: 172.
59. DelBene, E., Gatto, G., and Poggioni, M. (1984). "Clinical and Pharmacological Intervention in Flunarizine-Treated Migrainous Children," Collegium Internationale Neuro-psychopharmacologicum, 14th C.I.N.P. Congress, Florence, June 19-23, 1984. Abstract F48-51.
60. Caers, L. I. and Ferriere, G. (1985). Flunarizine in the prophylactic treatment of pediatric migraine, *J. Neurol. 232 (suppl)*: 160.
61. Bonuso, S., Di Stasio, E., Marano, E., Sorge, F., and Leo, A. (1988). Sublingual flunarizine: A new effective management of the migraine attack. A comparison versus ergotamine, *Headache, 26*: 227-230.
62. Chouza, C., Caamano, J. L., Aljanati, R., Scaramelli, A., De Medina, O., and Romero, S. (1986). Parkinsonism, tardive dyskinesia, akathisia, and depression induced by flunarizine, *Lancet*,
63. Meyboom, R. H. B., Ferrari, M. D., and Dieleman, B. P. (1986). Parkinsonism, tardive dyskinesia, akathesia, and depression induced by flunarizine, *Lancet*,
64. Steardo, L., Marano, E., Barone, P., Denman, D. W., Monteleone, P., and Cardone, G. (1986). Prophylaxis of migraine attacks with a calcium-channel blocker: Flunarizine versus methysergide, *J. Clin. Pharmacol., 26*: 524-528.
65. Nuyten, S. T. M. (1985). Comparative trial of flunarizine and pizotifen in the prophylaxis of migraine, *J. Neurol., 232 (suppl.)*: 219.
66. Worz, R. and Drillisch, C. (1983). Migrane-Prophylaxe durch einen Kalziumeintrittzblocker, *M.M.W., 125*: 711.

67. Cerbo, R., Cassachia, M., and Formisano, R., et al. (1986). Flunarizine-pizotifen single-dose double-blind crossover trial in migraine prophylaxis, *Cephalgia, 6*: 15-18.
69. Soyka, D. and Oestreich, W. (1987). "Therapeutic Effectiveness of Flunarizine and Propranolol in the Interval Therapy of Migraine," Presented at 3rd International Headache Congress, Florence, September 22-25.
70. Solomon, G. D. (1986). Verapamil and propranolol in migraine prophylaxis: A double-blind, crossover study, *Headache, 26*: 325.
71. Bussone, G., Baldini, S., D'Andrea, G., Cananzi, A., Frediani, F., Caresia, L., Milone, F. F., and Boiardi, A. (1987). Nimodipine versus flunarizine in common migraine: A controlled pilot trial, *Headache, 27*: 76-79.
72. Solomon, G. D. (1985). Comparative review of calcium channel blocking drugs in migraine, *Headache, 25*: 368-371.

6

Additional Pharmaceutical Agents Used in Migraine Prophylaxis

Arthur H. Elkind *Elkind Headache Center, Mount Vernon, and New York Medical College, New York*

INTRODUCTION

In the last 30 years, many agents have been proposed and tested and have found a role in migraine prophylaxis. While some of the drugs have been used widely, in some cases their use has decreased as their efficacy seemed less apparent with the passage of time. The adverse effects of some of these agents also have contributed to their limited role in prophylaxis. One drug, cyproheptadine, has been used since the early 1960s and established a small place in the prophylaxis of childhood migraine (1). Published studies with this drug are limited (2). Other antiserotonin compounds and ergotamine have been available and used as prophylactic agents. The large group of NSAIDs has found a growing role in migraine prevention. Aspirin is one of the oldest and most widely used drugs in this group.

The platelet antagonists are used for the prevention of certain cerebrovascular disorders and to prevent thromboembolism in patients with prosthetic heart valves. They have a limited role in migraine therapy. Classic and complicated migraine are examples of disorders where these agents may find limited use (3,4).

The categories of agents discussed in this chapter may be useful in migraine prevention. Overlap of categories will occur, since some compounds have multiple pharmacological properties and their mode of action in vivo may be complex. For completeness, agents of no apparent benefit and questionable value also are mentioned.

SEROTONIN ANTAGONISTS

Serotonin ($5-HT_1$ —5-hydroxytryptamine) has been studied intensively since its isolation and is thought to play a vital role as one of the biogenic amines involved in migraine pathogenesis (5). Serotonin and its products of metabolism were investigated; one such degradation product, 5-hydroxyindoleacetic acid, was found to be significantly increased during a migraine attack (6,7). It also was demonstrated that whole-blood serotonin diminished at the onset of a migraine attack and persisted at low levels during the attack (8). A significant proportion of migraine patients exhibited these changes. Serotonin demonstrates properties that may be pertinent to migraine symptomatology, including maintenance of extracranial vasoconstriction (9). The substance also is present in small percentages in the median raphe nuclei of the brain stem; it is an important neurotransmitter. About 10% of whole-body serotonin is in the platelets. The major portion of serotonin is located in the enterochromaffin cells of the gastrointestinal tract.

The actions and changes in serotonin levels thought to occur during migraine have led to the search for compounds that act on serotonin receptors as antagonists (10). The sought-after prophylactic compounds would act as serotonin blockers by occupying the receptor site normally occupied by serotonin. Knowledge of receptor sites for different biogenic amines has led to the development of beta-adrenergic blockers and specific histamine blockers.

Other Pharmaceuticals Used to Treat Migraine 129

Neuropharmacologists have been aware of more than one type of serotonin receptor. At present, there are thought to be three types of 5-HT receptors (11).

Methysergide

Methysergide is an effective antiserotonin agent (12). It was studied with placebo controls over an extended period of time and found to be effective for migraine prophylaxis (13). The drug was introduced in the United States during the early 1960s for the treatment of migraine headaches. It was found to be ineffective for the acute treatment of migraine, although it is a derivative of ergot. Methysergide maleate is 1-methyl-d-lysergic acid butanolamide. It is a congener of methylergonovine and of lysergic acid diethylamide (LSD). The compound is an effective antagonist of serotonin-induced vasoconstriction of smooth muscle in blood vessels and the intestine. It also inhibits serotonin-induced paw edema through a serotonin-antagonistic effect. Some dopaminergic effect can be demonstrated for methysergide, but less than for lisuride or d-LSD. Fozard postulates that the migraine-preventive drugs, including methysergide, have a common mechanism of action (14). The drugs propranolol, amitriptyline, chlorpromazine, cyproheptadine, and pizotifen have a single property of blocking serotonin responses at the 5-HT D-receptor sites. The newer nomenclature for serotonin receptor sites is designated as 5-HT_1, 5-HT_2, and 5-HT_3. Recently, drugs have been developed that have the ability to block different receptor sites and, most recently, 5-HT_3 receptor antagonists have been developed. It is believed that metaclopramide has 5-HT_3 receptor antagonist activity; for example, in preventing chemotherapy-induced vomiting (11). Humphrey (15) has described 5-hydroxytryptamine receptors and classified them, although he describes the difficulties in classification. Newer drugs with specific binding-site affinities have expanded our knowledge of serotonin and binding sites (16–18). Testing of newer pharmacological agents with serotonin-specific blocking properties may lead to more effective and safer agents in migraine therapy. It is of interest that 5-HT agonists also are under investigation in migraine. Methysergide's mechanism of preventing migraine is not definitely known.

In an early study with methysergide in 421 patients (13), the drug was found to reduce the frequency of headaches by at least 50% in 83% of the patients studied for more than two months. Overall, there was a 64% improvement in treated patients. There had to be a 50% reduction in headache frequency for treatment to be considered effective. Other investigators have demonstrated similar levels of effectiveness (19,20). A recent report (21) comments on the adequacy of earlier studies.

The dosage usually used varies from 2 to 8 mg per day in divided doses. The tablet is available in a 2-mg quantity. Because methysergide has been reported to increase gastric acidity, it is best administered with food or antacids. If symptoms suggest increased gastric-acid secretion, additional methods to buffer gastric contents or reduce gastric-acid secretion may be used. Within two or three days, reduced headache frequency and severity usually are noted. One approach is to start with 2 mg per day and gradually increase the dosage every third day by adding a tablet with each meal. If a response is not obtained with 8 mg per day, it is unusual for larger dosages to produce a desired effect. Many patients complain of adverse effects of a transient nature with the first dose. Specifically, chest, abdominal, or leg cramps; anxiety; feelings of unreality; and distortion of body image may occur initially and not recur after subsequent doses or diminish in intensity. The incidence of side effects is high and may include side effects other than those described. Gastrointestinal, mental, neurological, vascular, and musculoskeletal symptoms may occur. Weight gain also is reported. If adverse symptoms occur but diminish and subside completely, patients may be encouraged to continue treatment. Very often, a slow increase in dosage will permit an individual to continue with therapy, which is to be encouraged when a beneficial effect occurs. Persistence of adverse symptoms would warrant discontinuing treatment.

Peripheral vascular disease, severe hypertension, coronary artery disease, inflammatory venous disease of the extremities, and septic states are contraindications to the use of methysergide. It is

Other Pharmaceuticals Used to Treat Migraine

best avoided during pregnancy. Renal and hepatic disease also limits its use.

When the agent was initially introduced into clinical use, patients were on continuous prolonged therapy that exceeded six months, and retroperitoneal fibrosis with ureteral obstruction, hydronephrosis, and azotemia were noted (22). With long-term use without interrupted therapy, complications such as pleuropulmonary fibrosis and endocardial fibrosis with thickening of the cardiac valves also have been described (23). The fibrotic syndromes may develop without clinical signs or symptoms and may be detected only by radiographic studies, including intravenous urography. It also has been learned that interrupted therapy, with a methysergide holiday of two or three months following four to six months of treatment, will prevent its occurrence. The fibrotic disorders usually resolve after the drug is discontinued. However, cardiac fibrosis may persist.

Patients should be under a physician's continuous supervision while on therapy. At times, it may be difficult to wean a patient from treatment, but other prophylactic agents can help in many patients where an exacerbation is expected or occurs. Withdrawal of methysergide should be gradual to avoid an exacerbation of symptoms. Patients should not use excessive quantities of ergot-containing drugs during a weaning period and, if possible, should avoid them altogether.

Arterial insufficiency of the lower extremity is a rare complication of methysergide therapy. A recent review (24) categorizes two types of angiographic patterns in methysergide toxicity. First, intra-abdominal extrinsic compression of the aorto-iliac vessels is seen with retroperitoneal fibrosis. Second, a marked diffuse bilateral spasm of the superficial femoral arteries may occur. The spasm is unassociated with retroperitoneal fibrosis.

In one reported series, (25), it was concluded that patients with the fewest number of headaches and those with symptoms suggestive of a cerebral disturbance responded to the agent best. The agent probably is best reserved for patients who suffer clear-cut migraine with a frequency that warrants prophylactic therapy. It probably is not effective for those individuals with daily or near daily mixed-type headaches. It also is not of benefit in tension-type headaches.

Pizotifen

Pizotifen is a benzocycloheptathiophene derivative. It is structurally similar to cyproheptadine and the tricyclic antidepressants. It exerts antiserotonin and antihistamine properties with anticholinergic action. It also has been proposed that the agent may occupy serotonin-receptor sites and mimic its action (26). It is thought that the drug's serotonin-antagonist activity is related to its efficacy in migraine. Classic and common migraine have been reported to be responsive to its action (27,28). It reduces migraine frequency in some individuals (29-31). The drug is not available in the United States, but has been used in Europe and Canada.

Numerous controlled studies have been reported that demonstrate the effectiveness of pizotifen. Some clinical trials have not demonstrated effectiveness greater than placebo (32). It appears to be less effective than methysergide, but some patients who do not respond to methysergide may respond to pizotifen. Recent studies have shown an effectiveness equal to flunarizine (33) and nimodipine (34), both calcium-channel-blocking agents. Pizotifen also may have calcium-channel-blocking activity (35). It also has shown an effect equal to metoprolol in reducing migraine frequency (36). Metoprolol is a cardioselective beta-adrenergic-blocking agent. Pizotifen is ineffective in the acute treatment of migraine.

The usual therapeutic dosage of pizotifen is 1.5 to 3.0 mg per day. The drug has a plasma half-life of 22.6 hours, and it has been suggested that a single daily dose would be effective, particularly at bedtime. Drowsiness and weight gain are the most common adverse effects. Other side effects include nausea, dizziness, and dry mouth. Most studies indicate that the agent is well tolerated, though weight gain appears to be greater with pizotifen than with flunarizine, nimodipine, or metoprolol. Some investigators report that the adverse effects diminish with prolonged therapy. Retroperitoneal fibrosis and other fibrotic disorders have not been reported with pizotifen.

Cyroheptadine

Cyproheptadine has been available for over 20 years, principally as an antihistamine (H_1 antagonist) and also with antagonist properties to acetylcholine and serotonin (37). It has found limited usefulness in treating migraine, principally as a preventive and not for acute therapy. The dosage is from 4 mg per day to 16 mg per day, with an occasional patient tolerating a total dosage of 32 mg per day. Therapy is limited in adults by the drug's tendency to produce drowsiness. Weight gain frequently accompanies long-term usage. The agent occasionally is helpful in treating childhood migraine, which sometimes is associated with weight loss. The use of cyproheptadine often will improve appetite and cause weight gain, which is desirable with these children. Other side effects include anticholinergic symptoms of urinary retention and dry mouth. Very infrequently, agitation, confusion, and visual hallucinations may occur with its use.

In the United States, cyproheptadine is one of the few available serotonin antagonists, in addition to methysergide, that may decrease the frequency of migraine attacks. It also may be used by some women as a premenstrual migraine preventive. Dosages of 4 to 16 mg per day for three to four days before the onset of expected menstruation may reduce the incidence of menstrual-related migraine. There have been few controlled studies with cyproheptadine in migraine prophylaxis; however, the author has found the drug to be of benefit in an occasional patient.

Peroutka (38) believes that the primary action of cyproheptadine in preventing contractions of the canine basilar artery is antagonism of calcium channels. The action of this drug in migraine may be similar to that of other CCB agents that appear to be effective in migraine prophylaxis. Pizotifen may have a similar mechanism of action.

Femoxitine

Femoxitine is a selective inhibitor of 5-hydroxytryptamine reuptake. A trial was undertaken comparing the drug to propranolol 160 mg daily (39). Propranolol was observed to be more effective in reducing headache frequency. Partial depletion of thrombocyte 5-hydroxytryptamine did not lead to a marked improvement in migraine frequency. A second study in 1986 (40) also could not demonstrate a beneficial effect of the agent in prevention of migraine. Dosages were started at 200 mg and gradually increased to 600 mg daily.

In two randomized studies it could not be demonstrated that femoxitine had an effect on attack frequency or headache index. The authors of one study (40) hypothesized that platelet 5-HT2 is not of major importance in migraine pathogenesis. They stated the hypothesis is open to question on the basis of the femoxitine studies. More recent studies involving a serotonin agonist implicate this neurotransmitter.

Additional Serotonin Antagonists

Recent advances in developing specific serotonin-receptor antagonists have led to new insight into serotonin-receptor sites. Ketanserin belongs to the $5\text{-}HT_2$ group and has little antagonistic effect on $5\text{-}HT_1$ receptors. It currently is under investigation in the treatment of hypertension. Trials with this or similarly specific agents may have a role in migraine prophylaxis. Currently, investigations are in progress or are planned with other serotonin antagonists as prophylactic agents.

ANTIPLATELET AGGREGATING AGENTS

Drugs with antiplatelet properties became popular in migraine prophylaxis during the 1970s when work by Kalendovsky (41) and Deshmukh (42) was reported. Platelet abnormalities were demonstrated in some individuals with complicated migraine (43). Extension of their conclusions led investigators to consider platelet abnormalities as a prime event or an important precipitating event of migraine headache. Therefore, drugs with potent properties in blocking platelet aggregation were sought after. A recent review casts doubt on the hypothesis of migraine as a platelet disorder (44), although it is conceded that any theory of migraine pathogenesis must explain the large body of data regarding platelet

Other Pharmaceuticals Used to Treat Migraine

function and migraine. Different categories of agents will be described with varying approaches to interfering with platelet activity. Concurrent with migraine therapy, some advances have been made in treating cerebrovascular disorders that involve platelet thrombi and embolization. Treatment regimens that have demonstrated some effectiveness in cerebrovascular disease also have been applied to migraine prophylactic regimens. Of late, a description in the *British Medical Journal* (45) of a collaborative trial with antiplatelet agents reviewed 31 randomized trials for patients with a history of transient ischemic attacks, occlusive stroke, unstable angina, or myocardial infarction. Vascular mortality was reduced in 29,000 patients by 15%. This study also demonstrated a reduction in total vascular events of 25%. No significant difference was demonstrated between the effects of varying types of antiplatelet treatments.

Migraine therapy using antiplatelet agents may involve several pharmacological regimens. There is no conclusive evidence or confirmation by repeat studies, of any particular agent having significant effectiveness in migraine prophylaxis.

Aspirin

The most widely used antiplatelet agent is aspirin. It is readily available and safe. A small but contolled study (3) suggested that aspirin was an effective prophylactic agent in doses of 650 mg or two tablets per day. Another study (41) where aspirin was combined with dipyridamole suggested that they were an effective combination in prophylaxis. Aspirin in very small doses (40 to 80 mg) can inhibit thromboxane A_2 synthesis (46). Thromboxane A_2 is a potent vasoconstrictor and platelet activator. In larger doses, aspirin also will prevent synthesis of prostacyclin, which is a potent vasodilator and platelet inhibitor. Platelets cannot synthesize new protein, and aspirin will permanently inactivate platelet cyclooxygenase, thereby preventing the formation of thromboxane A_2. Thromboxane may be the agent in platelets that plays a role in migraine causation or at least in the cascade of events that culminate in a migraine attack. For this reason, very small doses of aspirin may be more effective in preventing migraine, because they will permit prostacyclin formation to continue, but interfere with thromboxane A_2 production. The anticipated result is a reduction in headache frequency.

In one study (47) with aspirin in low dosages of 160 mg a day, no benefit was obtained in reducing the number or severity of migraine attacks. High dosages of aspirin were believed to be effective by a general analgesic effect.

The usual precautions must be taken with aspirin. It should not be used even in small doses for migraine prevention in those individuals with a history of sensitivity, bleeding tendencies, or peptic ulcer disease. Acute erosive gastritis may occur in the absence of a peptic ulcer. There is no need to give aspirin more often than once every 24 hours, since it blocks platelet aggregation and thromboxane synthesis for at least that period of time.

Sulfinpyrazone

Sulfinpyrazone originally was introduced as a uricosuric agent and was found to have a platelet-inhibitory function. It is thought to prolong platelet survival in several thromboembolic disorders. Two hundred milligrams four times a day would be used. Gastrointestinal side effects occur in a significant percentage of patients. Hypersensitivity reactions have been reported.

Dazoxiben

Dazoxiben is an analog of imidazole. It selectively inhibits thromboxane synthetase, but is inactive as an inhibitor of prostacyclin synthetase (48). The drug is absorbed orally and inhibits thromboxane synthetase in a dose-related manner. There is some evidence that the precursors of thromboxane that are blocked are redirected to synthesize prostacyclin. The drug has been found to be of benefit in Raynaud's syndrome. Joseph and coinvestigators (49) reported beneficial results in a limited study with dazoxiben, but the short half-life requires frequent doses. It also has been noted that the concomitant administration of small doses of aspirin inhibits the accumulation of the fatty acid cyclooxygenase

Other Pharmaceuticals Used to Treat Migraine 137

reaction that occurs during inhibition of thromboxane synthesis. A possible regimen in migraine prophylaxis would include dazoxiben and small doses of aspirin; further clinical trials are certainly indicated with this newer agent. Another approach to prolong platelet survival would be to simulate prostacyclin (PGI_2) formation with phosphodiesterase inhibition, potentiate endogenous PGI_2, and stimulate its release from blood vessels. Several agents are under investigation for such action. Dipyridamole, which is described in the next section, has phosphodiesterase-inhibitory action.

Dipyridamole

This compound has been used widely in cardiac and cerebrovascular disease to prolong platelet survival. The action of this drug on platelets may be to interfere with their function. It may act by promoting the intracellular concentration of cyclic adenosine monophosphate (AMP) and increasing the effect of prostacyclin (PGI_2) (50). The agent usually is combined with aspirin to prolong platelet survival. In instances of complicated or recurrent classic migraine, it may have a role with aspirin. Low dosages of aspirin, 325 mg a day or less, with dipyridamole in dosages of 25 mg three or four times a day may be effective. Higher dosages may produce headache and signs of peripheral vasodilation.

NONSTEROIDAL ANTI-INFLAMMATORY AGENTS (NSAIDS)

Several of the compounds in this group have been investigated for use as migraine preventives. Current concepts in the pathogenesis of migraine postulate a sequence of events initiated within the brain stem, involving neurovascular structures and concerned with platelet aggregation and serotonin and prostaglandin release with sterile inflammation. Prostaglandin inhibitors such as the NSAIDs may interfere in several phases of the suspected chemical alterations and, conceivably, may prevent migraine attacks before their inception. In fact, numerous trials have been conducted with these agents. Some of the studies reveal significant prevention of migraine when compared against placebo and agents previously found to be effective in migraine prophylaxis. Aspirin, indomethacin, naproxen, ketoprofen, flufenamic acid, and tolfenamic acid all have been used for this purpose, with varying degrees of effectiveness.

Among the most important actions of the NSAIDs is the inhibition of prostaglandin synthesis. When the levels of prostaglandins in various tissues are reduced, the actions they mediate are effected. Pain, inflammatory changes, platelet agglutination, and vascular reactivity are influenced by prostaglandins. Arachidonic acid is transformed through a series of steps into thromboxane and prostacyclin, as well asother prostaglandins and leukotrienes. The enzyme cyclooxygenase acts as the catalyst for the production of prostaglandins from arachidonic acid. The prostaglandins are thought to interact with bradykinin, producing pain and inflammatory changes following tissue injury. Some NSAIDs inhibit the enzymes cyclooxygenase and lipoxygenase. With inhibition, the amounts of these potent prostaglandins produced are limited. Migraine prevention may require a decrease in prostaglandin production, which the NSAIDs bring about. Different NSAIDs have different sites of action and block different enzyme systems, as well as having differing half-lives in the human. The length of action may determine if the agent will be effective in migraine prevention.

Aspirin

Aspirin is discussed on page 138.

Indomethacin

A methylated-indole derivative available since 1963 for the treatmet of rheumatoid arthritis, indomethacin has been used for headache therapy because of the suspected inflammatory changes thought to occur in migraine. Except for isolated headache disorders, it has a very limited value in migraine prophylaxis. Most

Other Pharmaceuticals Used to Treat Migraine

headache clinicians reserve its use for prevention of exertional headache, which does not always occur in migraine sufferers, and instances of sharp, short-lived head pain syndrome (51). The latter syndrome includes "ice-pick-like headache", "jabs and jolts," and "needle-in-the-eye syndrome," as described by different clinicians. The explanation for indomethacin's effectiveness is not clear, but its effectiveness may be related to its potent anti-inflammatory and analgesic properties. It is a potent inhibitor of prostaglandin production. Its analgesic properties are distinct from its anti-inflammatory properties, and it has a peripheral and central effect. The CNS effects may be responsible for its effectiveness in the headache disorders described.

The usual dosage is 25 to 50 mg three times a day with meals or antacids. A prominent CNS side effect may be headaches over the frontal areas. Because of its frequent gastrointestinal as well as other CNS and hematopoietic side effects, patients should be observed closely with extended use of the drug.

Naproxen, Naproxen Sodium, Fenoprofen, and Ketoprofen

Numerous studies have appeared that describe these agents as prophylactic drugs in migraine therapy. They belong to the propionic acid derivative group, which also includes ibuprofen. They are usually tolerated better than other agents such as aspirin and indomethacin.

Naproxen, as well as other members of this group, still exhibits many of the harmful effects of other NSAIDs. It also has been noted that the short-acting agents are less likely to cause adverse effects (52). Patients who are intolerant of aspirin may have similar side effects with this compound. Gastrointestinal side effects may occur. Naproxen has a half-life of 14 hours in plasma and may be well suited for prophylaxis in migraine on a BID-dosage schedule. Dosages varied between naproxen 250 mg BID to 500 mg BID and naproxen sodium 550 mg BID. The studies (53,54) confirmed the effectiveness of the agents against placebo. In one study (55), propranolol was preferred by subjects and investigators as having been better tolerated with fewer gastrointestinal side effects. In another study (56), naproxen sodium 550 mg BID was equal in effectiveness to pizotifen 0.5 mg three times a day (TID). Both agents were used up to three months. Fenoprofen (57) in a dosage of 600 mg (TID significantly reduced headache frequency. Gastrointestinal side effects occurred in 13.5% of patients.

A study (58) using naproxen as a prophylactic agent in a dosage of 500 mg BID during a period of ergotamine withdrawal was found to be useful in reducing symptoms during this time. Further studies will be needed before a clear role for the propionic acid derivatives is established. Preliminary reports, however, suggest that they may play a useful role in migraine prophylaxis, and menstrual migraine may be particularly responsive to these agents.

Mefenamic Acid and Tolfenamic Acid

Both agents have been used in migraine therapy (59,60). Mefenamic acid was reported to be of benefit in premenstrual syndrome and helped to reduce headache symptoms by a signficant degree (61). Tolfenamic acid was reported to be of value in relieving the symptoms of withdrawal from ergotamine abuse (62). The drug was given in dosages of 200 mg TID, combined with chlordiazepoxide. Ergotamine abuse is a recognized disorder, and reports of tolfenamic acid and the previously mentioned naproxen used for prophylaxis in ergotamine withdrawal are encouraging. Many patients require mediation during the period of ergot elimination, and NSAIDs are reported to be of value.

Recent reports (63) emphasize the potentially harmful side effects of this group of seemingly safe compounds. Renal effects of NSAIDs can be prominent in individuals with preexisting renal disease, congestive heart failure, hypertension, and liver disease (64–66). Their use in chronic inflammatory disease of the small and large intestine also may result in an exacerbation of symptoms. It has been noted in a British study (52) that NSAIDs with longer plasma half-lives were associated with more toxic effects. Ibuprofen, with an elimination half-life of 1 to 2 hours, was associated with the least serious side effects, and piroxicam, with a 35-hour elimination half-life, had a much higher number of serious adverse side effects.

ERGOT ALKALOIDS
Ergotamine Tartrate

Ergotamine tartrate has been used for the treatment of migraine for many decades and has been the standard of therapy for the acute attack. Recent advances in the assay of ergot alkaloids enable one to determine ergotamine levels in plasma with radioimmunoassay and high-performance liquid chromatography. The compound is metabolized in the liver and excreted in the biliary system. Bioavailability varies, and some migraine sufferers using the drug on a daily basis in high dosage have a low frequency of serious side effects which may reflect its low bioavailability (67).

It has been suggested that the mode of action in migraine is by means of selective arterial vasoconstriction on certain cranial vessels or depression of central serotonergic neurons mediating pain transmission. Recent animal experiments (68) demonstrated that both ergotamine and dihydroergotamine act peripherally as competitive alpha-1-adrenoceptor antagonists and partial alpha-2-adrenoceptor agonists. Studies in humans (69) demonstrated no change in cerebral blood flow during intravenous administration of ergotamine or dihydroergotamine. Some work (70) suggests that ergotamine and related alkaloids have a common mechanism of action that enhances guanylate cyclase-cyclic GMP, which may explain their loss of effectiveness with chronic administration. Ergotamine is not an effective prophylactic agent and may lead to dependency.

Nitrate usage has several parallels to ergot administration. Nitrates have been found to be most effective when there is a pause in adminstration; otherwise, tolerance and loss of effectiveness develop (71,72). The lack of effectiveness is most noticeable with nitroglycerine in ointment or patch administration. Effectiveness is reestablished with a temporary cessation in usage. In other words, intermittent therapy is unassociated with tolerance. Nitrates also are involved in guanyl cyclase-cyclic GMP enhancement

(72,73) and possibly act by mimicking the vasodilating action of an endothelium-derived relaxing factor. The mechanism finally involves depletion of sulphydryl group donors. Further work (74) with ergotamine on isolated human superficial temporal artery reveals tachyphylaxis. A vasoconstrictive and 5-HT-blocking activity was demonstrated. Its beneficial effect may be interference during vasoconstriction and vasodilation in migraine.

As a rule, ergotamine tartrate is combined with other compounds for the relief of acute migraine. However, ergotamine tartrate as the sole agent is marketed in a sublingual form. It also is dispensed as an inhalation preparation. Some clinicians have attempted to use ergotamine tartrate as a preventive agent, with the use of a daily small oral dose. Before the introduction of agents with more demonstrable prophylactic action, it was used occasionally with a questionable degree of effectiveness.

Ergotamine can be abused easily, and a rebound-type headache may occur that precludes more widespread use. Ergotamine-rebound headache and abuse with dependency were well recognized in the 1950s (75). With recognition of the dangers and likelihood of dependency, most physicians avoid frequent use of ergotamine. Daily use certainly could be fraught with the risk of dependency as well as ergotism. Symptoms of ergotism may include acrocyanosis, acroparesthesias, intermittent claudication, nausea, and abdominal pain. In one review, it was felt by the authors that withdrawal of the agent was worthwhile, although there was a failure rate of 25%.

Small dosages on the order of 1 or 2 mg a day have been used orally and larger amounts by the rectal route for self-administered prophylaxis. There are a substantial number of patients who self-medicate with ergotamine tartrate on a daily basis. This regimen is not a deliberate trial of prophylaxis—it is a dependency problem in patients with many years of headache. Their withdrawal from ergotamine then is followed by rebound headache. Dependent individuals believe it is a prophylactic agent, because daily use diminishes the migraine-like morning rebound headache that is brought about by the repeated use of the agent. Ergotamine subdues the rebound headache until the drug is metabolized. As a

Other Pharmaceuticals Used to Treat Migraine

consequence of the dissipation of ergotamine tartrate, rebound migraine-like headache occurs. The rebound headache is mistaken for a migraine, and it may be a violent headache with some of the same features. Tfelt-Hansen and Olesen (76) reported on the arterial response to ergotamine tartrate in abusing as well as non-abusing patients. They could not demonstrate a hypersensitivity or tolerance to ergotamine in chronic abusers. They commented that previous abuse is a relative contraindication to its use, but if patients are not permitted a slow escalation in dosage, repeat abuse of the agent will not occur. Patients can be given ergotamine for acute migraine headache if they find it the only agent that will relieve their attacks. Dosages must be carefully controlled, and treatment with ergotamine must be limited to one course per week of 6 mg maximum.

A variation on the use of ergotamine tartrate is the same compound combined with belladonna and phenobarbital. The product is marketed in the United States as Bellergal-S® tablets. The exact formulation is phenobarbital 40 mg, ergotamine tartrate 0.6 mg, and levoratatory alkaloids of belladonna, as maleates, 0.2 mg. The phenobarbital is used for sedation, the ergotamine tartrate is a sympathetic inhibitor through its alpha-adrenergic-inhibiting action, and the belladonna acts as a parsympathetic-blocking agent. The usual dosage is 1 tablet BID. Bellergal-S® tablets are easily tolerated, with few serious adverse side effects. The usual contraindications and drug interactions are present for each of the components. The author has used the short-acting preparation since 1962. It was originally introduced in a short-acting form. The presently available preparation is a sustained-release tablet that permits a dose every 12 hours. It is effective in a limited number of migraineurs in preventing headache. It also can be given as a preventive of premenstrual migraine by starting one tablet BID four days premenstrually and continuing through the menstrual period. The preparation is well tolerated and can be a starting medication for preventive therapy in some migraineurs before embarking on other regimens and complex pharmacotherapy. An occasional patient will exhibit a gratifying response. Fortunately, the preparation when administered regularly BID does not lead to ergotamine dependency. It is best to avoid additional ergotamine tartrate for symptomatic use when the patient is receiving the described combination.

A study (77) in 1977 involved a double-blind comparison and placebo. A crossover design indicated a benefit in the prophylaxis of throbbing headache. The parallel design did not demonstrate a difference in treatment groups. However, in view of the absence of serious, frequent side effects, an initial trial for prophylaxis in patients with migraine is warranted. It is usually not effective in individuals with mixed headache of a daily nature, also referred to as chronic daily headache.

Ergotamine tartrate is contraindicated in pregnancy, toxic states, coronary artery disease, severe hypertension, peripheral vascular disease, arteriosclerosis obliterans, and thrombophlebitis of the extremities. Individuals with Raynaud's disease should not receive the agent. Renal or hepatic disease also may preclude its use.

Dihydroergotamine Mesylate

Semisynthetic derivatives of the ergot alkaloids have been developed. Chemical alteration has yielded dihydroergotamine by catalytic hydrogenation of the natural alkaloids. It is one of the compounds that is saturated in ring D of lysergic acid. It is similar in action to ergotamine, but has noticeably less emetic action. Dihydroergotamine has partial agonist action on alpha-adrenoceptors in veins (68). It is antagonist in many other blood vessels, smooth muscles, and the peripheral and central nervous systems with alpha-adrenoceptor activity. It also was found not to alter cerebral blood flow in humans (69). As with ergotamine tartrate, it enhances guanylate cyclase activity (70) and therefore may be more effective with interrupted administration. The development of a programmed-release form (microgranules in a capsule) and the attainment of satisfactory plasma levels when compared to an oral solution prompted numerous trials with a preparation for migraine prophylaxis. In one study, it was found to be 71% effective. It was unsatisfactory in tension-vascular headache. A series of further investigations (79,80) with timed-release dihydroergotamine confirmed the efficacy, bioavailability, and low incidence of side effects. Some reports (81) comment on its particular effectiveness in nocturnal and morning headache. One report (82) noted efficacy in preventing menstrual migraine. The preparation is not available in the United States at present. Timed-release dihydroergotamine capsules may offer an alternative prophylactic form of therapy in migraine.

SEROTONIN PRECURSORS

L-5-hydroxytryptophan was compared to methysergide in one study (83) and found to reduce intensity and duration of the attack. The improvement of patients was 75% for methysergide and 71% for 5-hydroxytryptophan. A double-blind, crossover study (84) with L-5-hydroxytryptophan also was made in childhood migraine. The results were confounded by a treatment crossover-period interaction. The study revealed no adverse effects in treated patients. Other studies have yielded contradictory results. One investigative group believed that contradictory results were obtained because treatment groups must be subdivided. It appears, at present, that L-5-hydroxytryptophan cannot be recommended as an effective therapy for migraine prophylaxis, and further studies may be warranted to help clarify the compound's status.

DOPAMINERGIC AGONISTS

Lisuride is one of the ergot alkaloids with high dopaminergic activity, and it was reported in one study (85) to be as effective as methysergide. In two other studies (86,87), the authors stated that it was superior to placebo. The agent does not have an established role in migraine prophylaxis at present.

Bromocriptine also has been reported (85) to have a prophylactic value in migraine. Bromocriptine is used primarily as an added agent for the treatment of Parkinson's disease and for hyperprolactinemia in certain situations. It cannot be recommended at present for migraine-preventive therapy.

MISCELLANEOUS AGENTS
Suloctidil

Periodically, reports appear of various agents having prophylactic benefit in migraine. Because of the natural history of migraine, episodes frequently will appear to decrease following administration of an agent. Careful placebo-controlled studies with statistical analysis are required before an agent can be considered for prophylaxis. A recent symposium (88) describes in detail problems with drug studies in migraineurs.

Suloctidil is 1-(4-isopropylthiophenyl)-2-n-octylaminopropanol and is a peripheral vasodilator, with other actions including inhibition of platelet aggregation. Suloctidil was reported in an open pilot study (89) using 600 mg daily for six weeks. Twenty-seven patients were studied. A good response was observed in seven and significant improvement was noted in eleven patients. Treatment was rated as ineffective or doubtful in nine patients. Ten patients reported mild adverse effects including weakness, somnolence, dizziness, and slight dyspepsia. One patient stopped treatment because of adverse effects.

Clonidine

Clonidine is an alpha$_2$-adrenergic agonist, but only a partial agonist, and its effect is dependent on norepinephrine concentrations at a particular site. It is available and marketed in Europe as a migraine preventive, but in the United States it is recommended for the therapy of hypertension. Several conflicting reports exist as to its efficacy in migraine (90,91). The agent has been used for drug withdrawal and may be of value for migraine prevention in patients under treatment for dependency on ergotamine or other abused substances. Patients who are receiving therapy for hypertension and concomitant migraine may be responsive to clonidine. Dryness of the mouth and sedation are reported as adverse effects in many patients. Dosages in the range of 0.1 to 0.4 mg may be effective for hypertension, but in migraine prophylaxis a small amount may be adequate. There is some evidence that smaller

Other Pharmaceuticals Used to Treat Migraine

quantities are effective, but larger amounts interfere with preventive action.

Captopril

Several reports from European investigators comment on the preventive action of captopril, and angiotensin-converting enzyme inhibitor in migraine. Published reports are awaited for confirmation of this drug's role in migraine therapy.

Cyclandelate

Cyclandelate is a vasodilator that has properties similar to those of papaverine and is reported (92) to be of value in migraine prophylaxis. Further studies are necessary to determine its role, if any, in migraine prophylaxis.

SUMMARY

Some of the pharmaceutical agents described in this chapter are among the drugs with the longest history of use in migraine. Methysergide, pizotifen, and cyproheptadine have been studied over 20 years and have a role in prophylaxis. The antiplatelet agents—aspirin, sulfinpyrazone, and dipyridamole—are available, particularly for frequent classic and complicated migraine. Recent reports of satisfactory prophylactic effect with other NSAIDs—notably, naproxen, which has been studied most frequently in migraine—is well worth a trial in some patients. Bellergal-S® tablets are safe and have been found to be effective in selected patients. They can be a suitable initial form of prophylaxis. Continued studies of efficacy with oral dihydroergotamine retard capsules, if demonstrated to be satisfactory, may lead to their introduction. Several pharmaceutical firms are presently investigating compounds with antiserotonin, antiplatelet, and CNS action that may offer hope for the migraine sufferer who requires drug intervention for prophylaxis.

TABLE 1 Interval Therapy of Migraine

	Migraine occurring 3 or more times a month or disabling attacks	Contraindication or failure of beta or calcium blockers or tricyclics		
No contraindication to ergot alkaloids				No contraindication to NSAIDs
Trial of ergotamine as Bellergal-S® daily	Methysergide Limit 4 to 6 months of continuous therapy	Pizotifen (if available) or cyproheptadine (nocturnal administration), childhood migraine	Trial with Aspirin (low dose) and dipyridamole	Propionic acid derivatives, as naproxen

TABLE 2 Selection of Interval Therapy with Additional Agents

Indicated drug	Special uses in complicated illness, contraindications to other drugs, or special indication
Clonidine	Hypertension; drug dependency
Bellergal-S	Peptic ulcer, salicylate sensitivity precludes NSAIDs
Aspirin and dipyridamole	Migraine with prolonged neurological symptoms and signs
	Vasospastic disorders, thromoembolism Raynaud's disease
Cyproheptadine	Presence of multiple medical illnesses: cardiac, diabetes, peptic ulcer; prophylaxis with need for weight gain
Methysergide	Severe clear-cut migraine attacks with refractory status to other agents
Naproxen	Menstrual migraine, well accepted

A practical approach to interval therapy is outlined for those patients where beta-adrenergic compounds cannot be used (Table 1). At times, patients cannot receive calcium-channel blockers or tricyclic antidepressants concomitantly. Migraine is a common disorder, and occasional patients are confronted with associated illnesses, contraindications, and special problems, yet they require prophylactic treatment; several compounds are listed with special indications (Table 2).

REFERENCES

1. Bille, B., Ludvigsson, J., and Sanner, G. (1977). Prophylaxis of migraine in children, *Headache, 17*: 61-63.
2. Lance, J. W. (1982) *Mechanism and Management of Headache* (4th ed.) Butterworth Scientific, London, p. 188.
3. O'Neill, B. P., and Mann, J. D. (1978). Aspirin prophylaxis in migraine, *Lancet, 2*: 1179-1181.

4. Masel, B. E., Chesson, A. L., Peters, B. H., Levin, H. S., and Alperin, J. B. (1980). Platelet antagonists in migraine prophylaxis. A clinical trial using aspirin and dipyridamole, *Headache, 20(1)*: 13-18.
5. Anthony, M., Hinterberger, H., and Lance, J. W. (1968). The possible relationship of serotonin to migraine, *Res. Clin. Stud. Headache, 2*: 29-59.
6. Curran, D. A., Hinterberger, H., and Lance, J. W. (1965). Total plasma serotonin, 5HIAA, and p-hydroxy-m-methoxymandellic acid excretion in normal and migraine subjects, *Brain, 88*: 997-1010.
7. Curzon, G., Theaker, P., and Phillips, B. (1966). Excretion of 5HIAA in migraine, *J. Neurol. Neurosurg. Psych., 29*: 80-85.
8. Anthony, M., Hinterberger, H., and Lance, J. W. (1967). Plasma serotonin in migraine and stress, *Arch. Neurol., 16*: 544-552.
9. Sicuteri, F. (1966).Vasoneuroactive substances in migraine, *Headache, 6*: 109-126.
10. Anthony, M. (1984). Serotonin antagonists, *Aust. NZ J. Med., 14(6)*: 888-895.
11. Anonymous (1987). 5-HT$_3$ receptor antagonists: A new class of antiemetics (editorial), *Lancet, 1*: 1470.
12. Fozard, J. R., (1975). The animal pharmacology of drugs used in the treatment of migraine, *J. Pharm. Pharmacol., 27(5)*: 297-321.
13. Friedman, A. P. and Elkind, A. H. Appraisal of methysergide in treatment of vascular headaches of migraine type, *JAMA, 184*: 125-128.
14. Fozard, J. R. (1982). Basic mechanisms of antimigraine drugs, *Headache*: *Physiopathological and Clinical Concepts* (M. Critchley, A. P. Friedman, S. Gorini, and F. Sicuteri, eds.), Raven Press, New York, p. 295.
15. Humphrey, P. P. (1984). Peripheral 5-hydroxytryptamine receptors and their classification, *Neuropharmacology, 23(12B)*: 1503-1510.
16. Leysen, J. (1984). Problems in in-vitro receptor binding studies and identification and role of serotonin receptor sites, *Neuropharmacology, 23(2B)*: 247-254.
17. Leysen, J. E., DeChaffoy DeCourcelles, D., DeClerck, F., Niemegeers, C. J. E., and VanNueten, J. M. (1984). Serotonin-S$_2$ receptor binding sites and functional correlates, *Neuropharmacology, 23(12B)*: 1493-1501.

Other Pharmaceuticals Used to Treat Migraine

18. Peroutka, S. J. (1984). 5-HT$_1$ receptor sites and functional correlates, *Neuropharmacology, 23(12B)*: 1487-1492.
19. Graham, J. R. (1964). Methysergide for the prevention of headaches. Experience in 500 patients over 3 years, *NEJM, 270*: 67-72.
20. Curran, D. A. Hinterberger, H., and Lance, J. W. (1967). Methysergide, *Res. Clin. Stud. Headache, 1*: 74-122.
21. Gaudet, R. J. and Kessler I. I. (1987). Transparently blinded trials of methysergide (letter), *NEJM, 316(5)*: 279-280.
22. Elkind, A. H., Friedman, A. P., Bachman, A., Siegelman, S. S., and Sacks, O. W. (1968). Silent retroperitoneal fibrosis associated with methsergide therapy, *JAMA, 206*: 1041-1044.
23. Graham, J. (1967). Cardiac and pulmonary fibrosis during methsergide therapy for headache, *Am. J. Med. Sci., 257*: 1-12.
24. Dorne, H. L. and Satin, R. (1986). Methysergide induced lower extremity arterial insufficiency, *J. Can. Assoc. Radiol., 37(3)*: 210-212.
25. Drummond, P. D. (1985). Effectiveness of methysergide in relation to clinical features of migraine, *Headache, 25(3)*: 145-146.
26. Speight, T. M. and Avery, G. S. (1972). Pizotifen (BC-105): A review of its pharmacological properties and its therapeutic efficacy in vascular headaches, *Drugs (Switzerland), 3(3)*: 159-203.
27. Bademosi, O. and Osuntokun, B. O. (1978). Pizotifen in the management of migraine, *The Practitioner, 220*: 325-326.
28. Carroll, J. D. and Maclay, W. P. (1975). Pizotifen in migraine prophylaxis, *Current Medical Research and Opinion, 3*: 68-71.
29. Heathfield, K. W. G., Stone, P., and Crowder, D. (1977). Pizotifen in the treatment of migraine, *The Practitioner, 218*: 328-430.
30. Hughes, R. C. and Foster, J. B. (1971). BC 105 in the prophylaxis of migraine, *Current Therapeutic Research, 13*: 63-68.
31. Capildeo, R. and Rose, F. C. (1982). Single-dose pizotifen, 1.6 mg Nocte®: A new approach in the prophylaxis of migraine, *Headache, 22(6)*: 272-275.
32. Gillies, D., Sills, M., and Forsythe, I. (1986). Pizotifen (Sanomigran®) in childhood migraine. A double-blind controlled trial, *Eur. Neurol., 25(1)*: 32-35.
33. Cerbo, R., Casacchia, M., Formisano, R., Feliciani, M., Cusimano, G., Buzzi, M. G., and Agnoli, A. (1986). Flunarizine-pizotifen single-dose

double-blind crossover trial in migraine prophylaxis, *Cephalalgia, 6(1)*: 15-18.
34. Havanka-Kanniainen, H., Hokkanen, E., and Myllyla, V. V., (1987). Efficacy of nimodipine in comparison with pizotifen in the prophylaxis of migraine, *Cephalalgia, 7(1)*: 7-13.
35. Peroutka, S. J., Banshart, S. B., and Allen, G. S. (1985). Calcium channel antagonism by pizotifen, *J. Neurol Neurosurg. Psychiatry, 48(4)*: 381-383.
36. Vilmins, S., Standnes, B., and Hedman, C. (1985). Metoprolol and pizotifen in the prophylactic treatment of classical and common migraine. A double-blind investigation, *Cephalalgia, 5(1)*: 17-23.
37. Anonymous (1978). Cyproheptadine (editorial), *Lancet, 1*: 367.
38. Peroutka, S. J. (1983). The pharmacology of calcium channel antagonists: A novel class of anti-migraine agents? *Headache, 23(6)*: 278-283.
39. Kangasniemi, P. J., Nyrke, T., Lang, A. H., and Petersen, E. (1983). Femoxetine—a new 5-HT uptake inhibitor—and propranolol in the prophylactic treatment of migraine, *Acta Neurol. Scand., 68(4)*: 262-267.
40. Orholm, M., Honore, P. F., and Zeeberg, I. (1986). A randomized general practice group-comparative study of femoxetine and placebo in the prophylaxis of migraine, *Acta Neurol. Scand., 74(3)*: 235-239.
41. Kalendovsky, Z. and Austin, J. H. (1975). Complicated migraine: Its association with increased platelet aggregability and abnormal coagulation factors, *Headache, 15*: 18-35.
42. Deshmukh, S. V. and Meyer, J. S. (1977). Cyclic changes in platelet dynamics and pathogenesis and prophylaxis of migraine, *Headache, 17*: 101-107.
43. Kalendovsky, Z., Austin, J., and Steele, P. (1975). Increased platelet aggregability in young patients with stroke, *Arch. Neurol., 32*: 13-20.
44. Joseph, R. and Welch, K. M. A. (1987). The platelet and migraine: A nonspecific association, *Headache, 27(7)*: 375-380.
45. Anonymous (1988). Secondary prevention of vascular disease by prolonged antiplatelet treatment. Antiplatelet trialists' collaboration, *Br. Med. J. (Clin. Res.), 296(6618)*: 320-331.
46. Weksler, B. B., Pett, S. B., Alonso, D., Richter, R. C., Stelzer, P., Subramanian, V., Tack-Goldman, K., and Gay, W. A. (1983). Differential

inhibition by aspirin of vascular and platelet prostaglandin synthesis in atherosclerotic patients, *NEJM, 308(14)*: 800.
47. Hosman-Benjaminse, S. L. and Bolhuis, P. A. (1986). Migraine and platelet aggregation in patients treated with low dose acetylsalicylic acid, *Headache, 26(6)*: 282-284.
48. Randall, M. J., Parry, M. J., Hawkeswood, E., Cross, P. E., and Dickinson, R. P. (1981). U-37248, a novel, selective thromboxane synthetase inhibitor with platelet antiaggregating and antithrombotic activity, *Thrombosis Res., 23*: 145-162.
49. Joseph, R., Steiner, T. J., Poole, C. J. M., Littlewood, J., and Rose, F. C. (1985). Thromboxane synthetase inhibition: Potential therapy in migraine, *Headache, 25(4)*: 204-207.
50. Mehta, J. (1983). Platelets and prostaglandins in coronary artery disease, *JAMA, 249(20)*: 2818.
51. Mathew, N. T. (1981). Indomethacin responsive headache syndromes, *Headache, 21(4)*: 147-150.
52. Adams, S. (1987). Nonsteroidal antiinflammatory drugs, plasma half-lives, and adverse reactions (letter), *Lancet, 2*: 1204-1205.
53. Lindegaard, K. F., Overlid, L., and Sjaastad, O. (1980). Naproxen in the prevention of migraine attacks. A double-blind placebo controlled crossover study, *Headache, 20(2)*: 96-98.
54. Johnson, E. S., Ratcliffe, D. M., and Wilkinson, M. (1985). Naproxen sodium in the treatment of migraine, *Cephalalgia, 5(1)*: 5-10.
55. Sargent, J., Solbach, P., Damasio, H., Baumel, B., Corbett, J., Eisner, L., Jessen, B., Kudrow, L., Mathew, N., Medina, J., Saper, J., Vijayan, N., Watson, C., and Alger, J. (1985). A comparison of naproxen sodium to propranolol hydrochloride and a placebo control for the prophylaxis of migraine headache, *Headache, 25(6)*: 320-324.
56. Behan, P. O. and Connelly, K. (1986). Prophylaxis of migraine: A comparison between naproxen sodium and pizotifen, *Headache, 26(5)*: 237.
57. Diamond, S., Solomon, G. D., Freitag, F. G., and Mehta, N. D. (1987). Fenoprofen in the prophylaxis of migraine: A double-blind, placebo controlled study, *Headache, 27(5)*: 246-249.
58. Mathew, N. T. (1987). Amelioration of ergotamine withdrawal symptoms with naproxen, *Headache, 27(3)*: 130-133.

59. Johnson, R. H., Hornabrook, R. W., and Lambie, D. G. (1986). Comparison of mefenamic acid and propranolol with placebo in migraine prophylaxis, *Acta Neurol. Scand., 73(5)*: 490-492.
60. Mikkelsen, B., Pedersen, K. K., and Christiansen, L. V. (1986). Prophylactic treatment of migraine with tolfenamic acid, propranolol, and placebo, *Acta Neurol. Scand., 73(4)*: 423-427.
61. Mira, M., McNeil, D., Fraser, I. S., Vizzard, J., nd Abraham, S. (1986). Mefenamic acid in the treatment of premenstrual syndrome, *Obstet. Gynecol., 68(3)*: 395-398.
62. Ala-Hurula, V., Myllyla, V. V., Hokkanen, E., and Tokola, O. (1981). Tolfenamic acid and ergotamine abuse, *Headache, 21(6)*: 240-242.
63. Garella, S. and Matarese, R. A. (1984). Renal effects of prostaglandins and clinical adverse effects of nonsteroidal anti-inflammatory agents, *Medicine, 63*: 165-181.
64. Ciabattoni, G., Cinotti, G. A., and Pierucci, A. (1984). Effects of sulindac and ibuprofen in patients with chronic glomerular disease: Evidence for the dependence of renal function on prostacyclin, *NEJM, 310*: 279-283.
65. Clive, D. M. and Stoff, J. S. (1984). Renal syndromes associated with nonsteroidal anti-inflammatory drugs, *NEJM, 310*: 563-572.
66. Blackshear, J. L., Davidman, M., and Stillman, M. T. (1983). Identification of risk for renal insufficiency from nonsteroidal anti-inflammatory drugs, *Arch. Int. Med., 143*: 1130-1134.
67. Perrin, V. L. (1985). Clinical pharmacokinetics of ergotamine in migraine and cluster headache, *Clin. Pharmacokinet., 10(4)*: 334-352.
68. Roquebert, J. and Grenie, B. (1986). Alpha 2-adrenergic agonist and alpha 1-adrenergic antagonist activity of ergotamine and dihydroergotamine in rats, *Arch. Int. Pharmacodyn. Ther., 284(1)*: 30-37.
69. Anderson, A. R., Tfelt-Hansen, P., and Lassen, M. A. (1987). The effect of ergotamine and dihydroergotamine on cerebral blood flow in man, *Stroke, 18(1)*: 120-123.
70. Vesely, D. L. (1983). Ergotamine and dihydroergotamine enhance guanylate cyclase activity, *Res. Commun. Chem. Pathol. Pharmacol., 40(2)*: 245-254.
71. Parker, J. O., Farrell, B., Lahey, K. A., and Moe, G. (1987). Effect of intervals between doses on the development of tolerance to isosorbide dinitrate, *NEJM, 316*: 1440-1444.

72. Cowan, J. C. (1986). Nitrate tolerance, *Int. J. Cardiol., 12*: 1-19.
73. Anonymous (1987). EDRF (editorial), *Lancet, 2*: 137-138.
74. Ostergaard, J. R., Mikkelsen, E., and Voldby, B. (1981). Effects of 5-hydroxytryptamine and ergotamine on human superficial temporal artery, *Cephalalgia, 1(4)*: 223-228.
75. Friedman, A. P. and Merritt, H. H. (1959). Migraine, *Headache: Diagnosis and Treatment* (A. P. Friedman and H. H. Merritt, eds.), F. A. Davis Co., Philadelphia, p. 241.
76. Tfelt-Hansen, P. and Olesen, J. (1981). Arterial response to ergotamine tartrate in abusing and nonabusing migraine patients, *Acta Pharmacologica et Toxicologica, 48(1)*: 69-72.
77. Stieg, R. L. (1977). Double-blind study of belladonna-ergotamine-phenobarbital for interval treatment of recurrent throbbing headache, *Headache, 17(3)*: 120-124.
78. Fontanari, D., Perulli, L., Conte, F., Tambato, E., Toso, V., and Zanetti, R. (1983). Planned release dihydroergotamine in common migraine and "tension-vascular" headache: Multicentre clinical trial, *Cephalalgia, 3 (Suppl. 1)*: 189-191.
79. Centonze, V., Attolini, E., Santoiemma, L., Brucoli, C., Macinagrossa, G., Campanozzi, F., and Albano, O. (1983). DHE retard for prophylactic therapy of migraine: Efficacy and tolerability, *Cephalalgia, 3 (Suppl. 1)*: 179-184.
80. Mastrosimone, F. and Iaccarino, C. (1983). Progress in migraine: Treatment with dihydroergotamine-retard, *Cephalalgia, 3 (Suppl. 1)*: 168-170.
81. Aylward, M., Chazot, G., Maddock, J., and Schott, B. (1984). Treatment of morning migraine. Clinical and biokinetic correlation of programmed-release dihydroergotamine, *Presse Med., 13(26)*: 1617-1619.
82. D'Alessandro, R., Gamberini, G., Lozito, A., and Sacquegna, T. (1983). Menstrual migraine: Intermittent prophylaxis with a timed-release pharmacological formulation o dihydroergotamine, *Cephalalgia, 3 (Suppl. 1)*: 156-158.
83. Titus, F., D'Avalos, A., Alom, J., and Ondina, A. (1986). 5-hydroxytryptophan versus methysergide in the prophylaxis of migraine. Randomized clinical trial, *Eur. Neurol., 25(5)*: 327-329.
84. Santucci, M., Cortelli, P., Rossi, P. G., Baruzzi, A., and Sacquena, T. (1986). L-5-hydroxytryptophan versus placebo in childhood migraine

prophylaxis: A double-blind crossover study, *Cephalalgia, 6(3)*: 155-157.
85. Horowski, R. (1982). Some aspects of the dopaminergic action of ergot derivatives and their role in the treatment of migraine, *Advances in Neurology. Headache: Physiopathological and Clinical Concepts* (M. Critchley, S. Gorini, A. P. Friedman, and F. Sicuteri, eds.) Raven Press, New York, p. 325.
86. Sommerville, B. W. and Herrmann, W. M. (1978). Migraine prophylaxis with lisuride hydrogen maleate—a double-blind study of lisuride versus placebo, *Headache, 18(1)*: 75-79.
87. DelBene, F., Poggioni, M., and Michelacci, S. (1983). Lisuride as a migraine prophylactic in children: An open clinical trial, *Int. J. Clin. Pharmacol. Res., 3(2)*: 137-141.
88. Rose, F. C., ed. (1987). Methodological problems in migraine trials, *Neuroepidemiology*, Karger, London, pp. 163-237.
89. Prusinski, A. (1983). Suloctidil therapy in migraine: An open pilot study, *Curr. Med. Res. Opin., 8(9)*: 631-633.
90. Boisen, E., Deth, S., Hubbe, P., Jansen, J., Klee, A., and Leunbach, G. (1978). Clonidine in the prophylaxis of migraine, *Acta Neurol. Scand., 58*: 288-295.
91. Mondrup, K. and Moller, C. E. (1977). Prophylactic treatment of migraine with clonidine: A controlled clinical trial, *Acta Neurol. Scand., 56*: 405-412.
92. Nappi, G., Sandrini, G., Savoini, G., Cavallini, A., deRysky, C., and Micieli, G. (1987). Comparative efficacy of cyclandelate versus flunarizine in the prophylactic treatment of migraine, *Drugs, 33 (Suppl. 2)*: 103-109.

7

Complicated Migraine and Migraine Equivalents

Donald J. Dalessio *Scripps Clinic and Research Foundation, La Jolla, California*

INTRODUCTION

The term *complicated migraine* usually is employed when the neurological manifestations that characterize migraine persist beyond the immediate headache period. Such neurological complications include hemiparesis, hemisensory defects, visual obscurations of various types, ophthalmoplegia, and related signs and symptoms. Most of these conditions are assumed to be due to prolonged vasoconstriction or vasodilation occurring as a part of the migraine syndrome. If the brain becomes ischemic enough during this vasoactive process, permanent damage may ensue or cerebral infraction may occur. Death has been reported in this situation, though probably this is a rare occurrence (1).

In this chapter, the following subjects will be discussed, which can be accommodated under the concept of hemiplegic migraine:

1. Migraine with prolonged aura
2. (Familial) hemiplegic migraine
3. Basilar migraine
4. Ophthalmoplegic migraine
5. Retinal migraine (ophthalmic migraine)
6. Migrainous infarction and migraine accompaniments

The incidence of complicated migraine is uncertain. The largest study, by Heyck and Krayenbuhl (2), reports on 980 patients with migraine, in whom they found an incidence of unilateral sensory signs in 3.8% and unilateral motor signs in 1.2%. These figures suggest that complicated migraine is a rare phenomenon. However, given the relative incidence of migraine in the general population, one may assume that complicated migraine probably occurs more often than has been reported previously.

MIGRAINE WITH PROLONGED AURA (MPA)

MPA occurs rarely. At least one aural symptom, often visual, should last for more than 60 minutes and less than 21 days (3–5). Full recovery should occur, as demonstrated by neurological exam and a study of the brain, either by computerized tomography (CT) or magnetic-resonance imaging (MRI) (6). If one of these studies shows evidence of a persisting vascular lesion, the diagnosis of migrainous infarction should be made (see below).

(FAMILIAL) HEMIPLEGIC MIGRAINE

Hemiplegic migraine illustrates the basic nature of the intracranial accompaniments of vascular headache of the migraine type (7). This variety of attack is accompanied by motor and sensory defects. Recovery usually is not prompt, and the hemiplegic signs and symptoms may persist for days or weeks, although complete recovery is usual. Such periods of motor and sensory defects may recur many times in the life span of the patient. Sometimes, the symptom complex occurs in families, with a strangely monotonous duplication of the clinical defects from person to person and

Complicated Migraine & Migraine Equivalents

in succeeding generations. This variety of attack may alternate with the more usual type of migraine, beginning with visual aura or simply with hemicrania and vomiting. Between attacks, there are no signs of impairment. The adjective *familial* has been placed in parentheses to emphasize that at least one first-degree relative should have identical attacks for this diagnosis to be made (8,9). But hemiplegic migraine is not always familial; the family history may be negative.

Alternating hemiplegia of childhood has been described and is related to migraine on clinical grounds (10). The hemiplegia occurs before 18 months of age, with repeated bilateral attacks. Other paroxysmal signs may include dystonias, autonomic disturbances, nystagmus, and tonic spells. Some researchers have suggested that alternating hemiplegia of childhood is an unusual form of epilepsy.

A recent report by Fitzsimmons and Wolfenden (11) describes a form of meningitic migraine with associated cerebral edema that also fits into the category of familial hemiplegic migraine. The family history in this report covered a period of 40 years. From this case study of seven patients, and from a review of the literature, the authors have concluded that familial hemiplegic migraine is an occasional cause of recurrent coma, which may be associated with life-threatening hemispheric edema, and that fever with CSF pleocytosis may occur. They also suggest that cerebral angiography is dangerous in this condition and may exacerbate coma and edema. In the family reported, cerebellar ataxia was present during recovery from attacks of hemiplegic migraine. Eventually, permanent cerebellar atrophy occurred, as demonstrated by CT scans.

BASILAR MIGRAINE

Basilar migraine (BM) is defined as migraine with aural symptoms that originate from the brain stem or from both occipital lobes (12). Usually, visual symptoms occur in both eyes, with associated dysarthria, vertigo, tinnitus, decrease in hearing, diplopia, ataxia, and bilateral alteration in motility or sensation (13). Decreased levels of consciousness may ensue.

Bickerstaff (12) studied 34 patients whose clinical symptoms also suggested involvement of the basilar system. All were under age 35; all but two were under age 23. Twenty-six were adolescent girls. A history of migraine in close relatives was obtained in 28 cases.

The first symptom usually was visual. In some patients, this consisted of total loss of vision; in others, it involved simple visual images throughout both visual fields, usually so intense as to obscure vision. This was followed by vertigo, ataxia of gait, dysarthria, and, occasionally, tinnitus—not neccesarily in that order, and the ataxia was not necessarily associated with vertigo. Sensory manifestations consisted of tingling or numbness in both hands and feet and sometimes around both lips and on both sides of the tongue. These symptoms lasted from 2 minutes to a maximum of 45 minutes and then subsided rapidly, though if there had been complete loss of vision, symptoms dwindled more gradually (5 minutes) through a period of graying of vision. In each instance, the premonitory symptoms were followed by severe throbbing headache, usually in the occipital region, and often accompanied by vomiting. The headache finally ended when the patient slept. These attacks were infrequent, but commonly occurred with menstruation in the girls. Between attacks, many patients had more typical attacks of migraine. Over the years, the more bizarre features described above gradually waned.

Swanson and Vick (14) have reported their experience with 12 patients considered to have basilar migraine. They found this to be a distinctive disorder characterized by symptoms referable to dysfunction of brain-stem structures, in conjunction with more typical migraine phenomena. They describe in detail one patient in whom an attack of basilar migraine was captured by the EEG recording and appeared as a typical photoconvulsive episode. On several occasions, this patient became unconscious without warning. She had two attacks in a brightly lit environment while she was standing at the foot of an upward-moving escalator. In each episode, she suddenly lost vision and then quickly became unconscious for about three minutes, slumping in an akinetic fashion to the floor. Subsequently, during photic stimulation and EEG recording, she had an attack similar to those described above. The investigators made the point that approximately half of their patients with basilar migraine responded to anticonvulsant drugs. They discussed the possible relationships between basilar migraine and epilepsy, but drew no specific conclusions.

Sturzenegger and Meienberg (15) have recently reviewed their extensive experience with this diagnosis. They surveyed 89 patients in whom BM was suspected and, using rigorous criteria, were able to confirm the diagnosis in 49 patients (32 women, 17 men).

In the 49 patients with definite BM, the age of onset ranged from 10 to 62, 65% of them having their first attack in the second or third decade. Forty percent had BM attacks only, while 60% had other types of migraine attacks as well. A typical pattern of attacks, with an ischemic aura followed by predominantly occipital headache, was found in only 57%. The most frequent ischemic symptom was bilateral visual impairment (86%). Symptoms and signs of brain-stem dysfunction were vertigo (63%), gait ataxia (63%), bilateral paresthesia (61%), bilateral weakness (57%), and dysarthria (57%). Seventy-seven percent of the cases had disorders of consciousness (mainly syncope, confusion, and prolonged amnesia). Four patients (8%) had epileptic seizures during the migraine attacks. Seventy-three percent had a family history of migraine and 12% of epilepsy. EEGs were always abnormal during the attacks, with predominantly localized or generalized, mostly paroxysmal, slow wave activity. CT scans were normal except for two women with repeated BM attacks, who were smokers and taking contraceptive drugs and who, during an attack, experienced a cerebellar and an occipital lobe infarction, respectively.

OPHTHALMOPLEGIC MIGRAINE

In ophthalmoplegic migraine, repeated attacks of headache associated with paresis of one or more ocular cranial nerves occurs, in the absence of a demonstrable intracranial lesion (16). Paresis may involve one or more of the cranial nerves III, IV, and VI, in association with persisting headache. There should be normal CSF and anatomical studies (CT, MRI, or both), including views of the orbits. The condition is rare, and the literature is replete with isolated case reports, including a recent example (17). Nonetheless, this diagnosis has an old and remarkable history.

Elliot (18), in reviewing the subject, quoted Charcot's definition of ophthalmoplegic migraine as migraine associated with a third or other ocular nerve palsy, which is transient at first, but later may become permanent. The syndrome occurs in persons of all ages. Patients as young as 3 and as old as 70 years of age have been described.

Ophthalmoplegic symptoms, according to Riley (19), may develop in a patient who has had migraine headaches for many years; 50 years may intervene between the occurrence of the first migraine headache attack and the paralysis of the eye muscles.

The ache of ophthalmoplegic migraine is experienced behind or over the eye. It usually is confined to one side of the head and on the same side as the ophthalmoplegia. Occasionally, the headache is bilateral. When the duration of the headache is prolonged, or when the pain is very intense, nausea and vomiting occur. Vertigo may be associated with the headache. In addition to the headache, the usual preheadache visual disturbances of migraine may occur, including spots before the eyes and homonymous field defects but these are not relevant to this discussion.

The headache usually precedes the extraocular paralysis, the latter appearing 6 to 10 hours after the onset of the headache or with the subsidence of the attack. More rarely, from 1 to 10 days may elapse between the onset of a long-lasting headache and the palsy. The third, fourth, sixth, or portions of the fifth cranial nerves may be involved. Occasionally, all of them may be involved, presenting a complete external ophthalmoplegia.

In patients who have repeated attacks, it is usual for the paralysis to be transient in the earlier ones, with complete recovery; but later, the paralysis may persist for a few days to many months, with certain palsies ultimately becoming permanent.

When a patient is seen with an ocular palsy for the first time, it is difficult to choose between structural disease, including intracranial aneurysm, and ophthalmoplegic migraine. When such palsies are numerous, are short-lived, and recur over a period of years, there need be no such difficulty in diagnosis.

RETINAL MIGRAINE

This is a form of monocular (or binocular, rarely) scotoma or blindness that lasts less than one hour and that may (or may not) be associated with headache. At least one paper (20) describes the changes in retinal circulation of the eye involved, using fluorescein antiography and fundus photography, in a patient with cluster headache.

In another report (21), after years of episodic monocular visual loss, presumed to be migraine, two patients suffered persisting loss of vision from retinal vascular occlusion. One was a 34-year-old woman with systemic lupus who showed disease of both arterial and venous circulations. The other, a 62-year-old hypertensive man, had a central retinal vein occlusion. This report emphasizes the multiple factors that produce vascular retinopathy in migraine.

Hedges (22) has described a group of patients with isolated ophthlamic migraine. These are visual abnormalities occurring in patients over age 50, many of whom (one third) had a history of migraine, now quiescent. They may have single or recurring scintillating scotomata that may be homonymous and are not followed by headache. These patients had a relatively benign prognosis. A subgroup had monocular visual changes, and in this subset, almost half proved to have vascular disease. I suspect that many were describing amaurosis fugax; it reinforces the concept that monocular visual loss often is atheroembolic in origin and must be so considered by the treating physician.

Thus, these patients with retinal migraine require the most thorough ophthalmological and cerebrovascular investigations, with normal eye exams outside of an attack, and negative studies for embolism.

MIGRAINOUS INFARCTION AND MIGRAINE ACCOMPANIMENTS

We owe interest in this topic particularly to the efforts of C. Miller Fisher (23), whose observations deserve careful review and consideration. His patients presented with episodic transient visual and other neurological symptoms, but when investigated, embolic phenomena and occlusive vascular disease could not be demonstrated. Fisher believes, therefore, that these episodes are migrainous accompaniments of later adult life, occurring without headache—hence the term *transient migrainous accompaniments* (TMAs).

A reliable sign of migrainous paresthesias is the "march" of numbness as it gradually spreads over the face or fingers and hands and migrates from face to limb, or vice versa, or crosses to the face and hand on the opposite side. This evolution may last for 30 minutes, but commonly lasts 15 to 25 minutes. This gradual spread is unusual in thrombotic or embolic cerebrovascular disease. Pure sensory stroke due to thalamic ischemia is the only stroke whose evolution may resemble the typical march of migraine paresthesias, but this occurs only very rarely. Conversely, the march of sensory seizures is much more rapid, being measured in seconds.

The occurrence of two or more episodes, particularly if they closely resemble one another, is important in the diagnosis. This history helps to exclude cerebral embolism, which is a prime diagnostic possibility when there is only one attack. The history of a similar spell, as long as 20 to 30 years before, also is evidence for migraine. An identical vascular spell or series of spells, occurring years ago, also favors migraine over thrombotic vascular disease. The time between episodes varies widely.

The duration of the episode also may be of importance in the diagnosis. Classically, migrainous episodes last 15 to 20 minutes or longer, whereas most transient ischemic attacks last less than 15 minutes.

Other points of value in the diagnosis of transient migraine equivalents are the benign nature of the spell in retrospect and the rarity of permanent sequelae. Repeated good recovery from what appears initially to be a threatening situation is evidence for migraine. In Fisher's series, there were no permanent deficits. Fisher stressed further the importance of a normal arteriogram and the absence of a source of emboli as prerequisites for establishing the diagnosis of TMA. Where atherosclerotic plaque and migraine coexist, the diagnosis becomes more difficult, and the judgment depends on the experience and expertise of the clinician.

Yet, clinical observations suggest that the degree of cerebral vasospasm that occurs in classic migraine is more severe and asymmetrical than is generally appreciated. There are only a few pictures of migrainous vasospasm demonstrated angiographically, but those that are available are impressive. The latest, published by Lieberman et al. (24), describes a 39-year-old female with a history of migraine who developed bilateral cervical carotid and intracranial vasospasm during a migraine attack. This patient was entirely well and had no history of heart disease, diabetes, hyperlipidemia, or problems with her neck. Her only medication before admission consisted of acetaminophen. She was not taking ergot compounds, amphetamines, illicit drugs, or oral contraceptives, and there was no history of smoking. The right common carotid arteriogram, performed the day after the patient developed hemiplegic migraine, using the digital-subtraction imaging technique, demonstrated a complete occlusion of the cervical portion of the right internal carotid artery approximately 3 cm distal to the common carotid bifurcation. The next day, the right common carotid artery was open, but there was decreased caliber of the cervical internal carotid artery and narrowing of the proximal segment of one of the branches of the right middle cerebral artery. At this time, also, the left common carotid artery demonstrated focal narrowing involving the left cervical internal carotid artery.

Similar related observations have been published sporadically over the last 20 years. One should not ignore these observations or the striking hemispheric changes in blood flow that have been reported by others. It is clear that, at least in some patients with migraine, there are marked vasospastic alterations in intracranial blood flow that are, for the most part, benign and that leave no residual neurological abnormality.

Finally, an occasional patient with complicated migraine will have a permanent neurological deficit and presumably has suffered a vasospastic stroke (25,26). Here, the boundary between benign vasospasm (migraine) and stroke would seem to have been completely erased.

This leads naturally to the concept of migrainous infarction. One relies on anatomical studies (CT, MRI, or both) to demonstrate hypodensity consistent with infarction in a patient with one or more migrainous auras that are not fully reversible. Again, other causes of infarction must be ruled out by careful anatomical investigation and study. Even then, the precise relationship between migraine and infarction is tenuous; an increased risk for stroke in migraine patients has not been found in carefully conducted epidemiologic surveys.

TREATMENT OF COMPLICATED MIGRAINE

Fortunately, as emphasized above, complicated migraine is uncommon. Treatment of complicated migraine is itself a complicated subject. I advise avoidance of vasoconstrictors, including all members of the ergotamine family. Although it never has been shown that ergot compounds produce intracranial vasoconstriction, that possibility exists theoretically; hence, this admonition.

Generally, one needs to educate the patient regarding risk factors that can be avoided. These include foods containing vasoactive substances, alcohol, cigarette smoking, and some medications, including estrogens. Hypertension, if present, must be controlled.

If these things are done, and if attacks continue, prophylactic preventive therapy should be employed. Beta blockers can be used in standard dosages. At least four—including propranolol, nadolol, timolol, and metoprolol—have been demonstrated to be effective in migraine in double-blind studies (27–30), though not specifically in complicated migraine.

Calcium-channel blockers (CCB) may prevent cerebral vasospasm or vascular overactivity and would appear to offer theoretical advantages in the treatment of complicated migraine. The CCBs affect the influx of calcium into vascular smooth muscle and so alter the ability of vessels to constrict. Although they may, therefore, be perceived as vasodilators, their ability to alter excessive vasomotor reactivity at least provides a theoretical basis for their use in the prophylaxis of migraine. Some CCBs are selective for intracerebral, as opposed to peripheral, blood vessels.

Preliminary studies have established that several of these compounds, including nimodipine, nifedipine, verapamil, flunarizine, and cinnarizine, are effective in headache prophylaxis. In addition, other drugs known to be useful in headache prophylaxis, including cyproheptadine and amitriptyline, have been shown to have significant calcium-antagonistic properties and can be considered as nonspecific CCBs.

In a recent case report (31), Goldner and Levitt describe the treatment of complicated migraine in a young woman, employing sublingual nifedipine 10 mg, given once only. This drug can be employed on a prophylactic basis or used at headache onset if attacks are infrequent.

A second case report (32), employing flunarizine in hemiplegic migraine, achieved similar results. Flunarizine also is reported as effective in alternating hemiplegia of childhood (33). Unfortunately, this medication is not available in the United States.

Further study of CCBs in complicated migraine is clearly indicated.

MIGRAINE EQUIVALENTS

Not all migrainous events of a complex nature fit easily into the category of complicated migraine. What remain are clinical impressions of so-called migraine equivalents, or migraine without headache, presumably manifested in other manners, in distant sites, often including pain (34).

Thus, migraine equivalents are defined as paroxysmal recurrent symptom complexes characterized by the following:

1. No demonstrable organic lesion
2. Previous history of typical migraine headache
3. Replacement of headaches by the equivalent syndrome
4. Absence of symptoms between attacks
5. Family history of migraine
6. Relief from the equivalent syndrome using appropriate drugs

Migraine equivalents may take several forms, including abdominal, ophthalmic, psychic, and autonomic (34).

Abdominal migraine is characterized by recurrent episodes of vomiting and/or abdominal pain in association with symptoms of the migraine attack. It is the most common visceral manifestation of migraine. Although it has been reported in patients from infancy to old age, it is most common between the ages of 2 and 11 years, and males are most often affected. Abdominal migraine often is characterized by a prodromal period of yawning, listlessness, drowsiness, or the typical aura of the migraine attack. The episode usually starts suddenly and is precipitated by a specific or stressful experience. The pain may be situated anywhere in the abdomen, but is usually epigastric or periumbilical. The individual bout of pain varies in severity, usually lasting one to six hours, and frequently is characterized by severe nausea and vomiting. There also may be a typical headache, constipation or diarrhea, lethargy, stuporous sleep, or irritability associated. Electroencephalography performed during the attack may show a mild generalized dysrhythmia.

Ophthalmic (retinal) migraine has been discussed above. Sometimes termed *acephalgic migraine*, it must be differentiated from amaurosis fugax, which implies atheromatous disease. Ophthalmic migraine is more properly considered as a form of complicated migraine, in the author's opinion, and hence its inclusion in the previous section.

Psychic migraine is probably more common than realized and is characterized by transient mood disorders or psychotic states that replace a typical unilateral headache. Often, there is a short prodromal period of lethargy or vigor, followed by a mood disorder lasting from a few hours to days. Many patients experience similar symptoms before a typical migraine attack, but in psychic migraine no headache occurs.

Various autonomic dysfunctions are common in patients with migraine. These include Raynaud's phenomenon, flushing, and even, on occasion, hemorrhage into the skin. Recurrent febrile episodes as a migraine equivalent have been reported.

TREATMENT OF MIGRAINE EQUIVALENTS

Often, no specific therapy is required beyond reassurance and education. If the migraine-equivalent syndrome becomes more chronic—for example, abdominal migraine—then a therapeutic trial using the usual preventive medications, such as beta blockers, can be employed.

SUMMARY

The concept of complicated migraine has been defined, and six separate types have been discussed. (There may be more.) Complicated migraine blends into classic migraine at times and abuts against frank cerebral infarction. It may be related to some unusual forms of epilepsy. Nonetheless, with attention to the history and examination, and by employing modern neurological investigations, it should be possible for the clinician to establish a working diagnosis in most situations of complicated migraine and to further subdivide the topic by type.

Treatment usually will be prophylactic or preventive. The calcium-channel blockers are the drugs of choice in this situation.

Migraine equivalents are related phenomena, a type of migraine without headache, manifested elsewhere, often in distant sites and often characterized by local pain. Several types are described that are derived from clinical impressions, and treatment is discussed briefly.

REFERENCES

1. Guest, A. A. and Woolf, A. M. (1964). Fatal infarction of the brain in migraine, *Brit. Med. J. 1*: 225-227.
2. Heyck, H. and Krayenbuhl, H. (1964). *Der Kopfschmerz*, George Theieme/Verlag, Berlin.
3. Heyck, H. (1973). Varieties of hemiplegic migraine, *Headache, 12*: 135-142.

4. Holub, V., Chrast, B., and Saxl, O. (1965). Complicated migraine, *Kinderaerztl Prax, 33*: 539-546.
5. Pearce, J. M. and Foster, J. B. (1965). An investigation of complicated migraine, *Neurology, 15*: 333-340.
6. Tinuper, P., Cortelli, P., Sacquegna, T., and Sugaresi, E. (1985). Classic migraine attack complicated by confusional state: EEG and CT study, *Cephalgia, 5*: 63-68.
7. Bradshaw, P. and Parsons, M. (1965). Hemiplegic migraine, *Quart. J. Med., 34*: 65-86.
8. Blau, N. J. and Whitty, C. W. M. (1955). Familial hemiplegic migraine, *Lancet, 2*: 1115-1116.
9. Staehelin-Jensen, T., Olivarius, B., Kraft, M., and Hansen, H. (1981). Familial hemiplegic migraine. A reappraisal and long-term follow-up study, *Cephalgia, 1*: 33-39.
10. Kraegeloh, I. and Aicardi, J. (1980). Alternating hemiplegia in infants: Report of five cases, *Dev. Med. Child Neurol., 27*: 6-44.
11. Fitzsimmons, R. B. and Wolfenden, W. H. (1985). Migraine coma. Meningitic migraine with cerebral edema associated with a new form of autosomal dominant cerebellar ataxia, *Brain 108: 555-577.*
12. Bickerstaff, E. R. (1961). Basilar artery migraine, *Lancet, 1*: 15-17.
13. Bickerstaff, E. R. (1986). Basilar artery migraine, *Handbook of Clinical Neurology* (F. C. Rose, ed.), Elsevier Amsterdam, pp. 135-140.
14. Swanson J. W. and Vick, N. A. (1978). Basilar artery migraine, *Neurology, 28*: 782-786.
15. Sturzenegger, M. H. and Meienberg, O. (1985). Basilar artery migraine: A follow-up study of 82 cases, *Headache, 25*: 408-415.
16. Bickerstaff, E. R. (1964). Ophthalmoplegic migraine, *Rev. Neurol., 110*: 582-588.
17. Busson, G., LaMantia, L., Grazzi, L., et al. (1987). Internal ophthalmoplegia in complicated migraine: A case report, *Headache, 27*: 489-490.
18. Elliott, A. J. (1940). Ophthalmoplegic migraine, *Can. Med. Assoc. J., 43*: 242-244.
19. Riley, H. A. (1932). Migraine, *Bull. Neurol. Inst. NY, 2*: 429-450.
20. Kline, L. B. and Kelly C. B. (1980). Ocular migraine in a patient with cluster headaches, *Headache, 20*:253-257.
21. Coppeto, J. R., Lessell, S., Sciarra, R. S., and Bear, L. (1986). Vascular retinopathy in migraine, *Neurology, 36*: 267-270.

22. Hedges, T. R. (1980). An ophthalmologist's view of headache, *Headache, 20*: 253-257.
23. Fisher, C. M. (1980). Late-life migraine accompaniments as a cause of unexplained transient ischemia attacks, *Can. J. Neurol. Sci., 7*: 9-17.
24. Lieberman, A. N., Jonas, S., Hass, W. K., et al. (1984). Bilateral cervical carotid and intracranial vasospasm causing ischemia in a migrainous patient: A case of "diplegic migraine," *Headache, 24*: 245-248.
25. Boisen, E. (1975). Strokes in migraine: Report on seven strokes associated with severe migraine attacks, *Dan. Med. Bull., 22*: 100-106.
26. Bousser, M. G., Baron, J. C., Iba-Zizen, T., Comar, D., Cabanis, E., and Castaigne, P. (1980). Migrainous cerebral infarction: A tomographic study of cerebral blood flow and oxygen-extraction fraction with the oxygen-15 inhalation technique, *Stroke, 11*: 145-148.
27. Diamond, S. and Medina J. (1976). Double-blind study of propranolol for migraine prophylaxis, *Headache, 16*: 24-27.
28. Ryan, R. E., Sr., Ryan, R. E., Jr., and Sudilovsky, A. Nadalol: Its use in the prophylactic treatment of migraine, *Headache, 23*: 26-31.
29. Tfelt-Hansen, P., Standnes, B., Kangasniemi, P., Hakkarainen, H., and Olesen, J. (1984). Timolol vs. propranolol vs. placebo in common migraine prophylaxis—a double-blind multicenter trial, *Acta Neurol. Scand., 69*:1-9.
30. Steiner, T. J., Joseph, R., Hedman, C., and Rose, F. C. (1988). Metoprolol in the prophylaxis of migraine: Parallel-groups comparison with placebo and dose-ranging follow-up, *Headache, 28*: 15-23.
31. Goldner, J. A. and Levitt, L. P. (1987). Treatment of complicated migraine with sublingual nifedipine, *Headache, 27*: 484-486.
32. Tobita, M., Hino, M., Ichikawa, N., et al. (1987). A case of hemiplegic migraine treated with flunarizine, *Headache, 27*: 487-488.
33. Casaer, P. and Azou, M. (1984). Flunarizine in alternating hemiplegia in childhood, *Lancet, 2*: 579.
34. Catino, D. (1965). Ten migraine equivalents, *Headache, 5*: 1-11.

8

Management of Migraine in the Elderly

John Edmeads *University of Toronto, Toronto, Ontario, Canada*

INTRODUCTION

As many of our elderly patients tell us, "Everything changes when you get old." To a degree, this applies to headache. In terms of etiology, the clinician has to confront a somewhat different array of diagnostic possibilities in the septuagenarian than in the 20- or 30-year-old. This, in turn, calls for a somewhat different investigational approach, with more ready recourse to the laboratory and to imaging procedures to identify the more frequent instances of biochemical or structural lesions that accompany old age. Even when the elderly patient is found to have the same sort of migraine or tension headaches that afflict those who are younger, the treatment may be different, because older people tend to have more incidental disease than younger people, with more potential contraindications and more potential side effects.

Defining old age is always a hazardous business, but quite arbitrarily and for this discussion, we shall consider it to be above the age of 60.

WHAT KINDS OF HEADACHES DO THE ELDERLY HAVE?

While there is no doubt that the benign functional headaches that begin in youth (migraine headache, tension headache, and cluster headache) tend to lessen with age (1), they still are a problem in the elderly. Largely, this is because there is, over the age of 50, a population of people who have not had the good fortune to be relieved of their headaches by advancing years. To a lesser but still perceptible extent, there are some patients who have had the onset of migraine, tension, or cluster headaches after the age of 50.

How large is the headache problem in the elderly? One epidemiologic technique, population surveys, goes out into the community and actively seeks out people with headache; this technique may overestimate the problem, since it usually gathers in those with all degrees of headache. In one of the better such surveys, Waters (2) found that 53% of males and 66% of females over the age of 55 had experienced headaches in the previous year; and 22% of males and 55% of females over the age of 75 had suffered headaches. This contrasted with prevalence rates of 74% for males and 92% for females in the age group from 21 to 34. Thus, while the headache problem seems to lessen with age, clearly it does not disappear.

Another epidemiologic technique records the number of physician services rendered or numbers of patients seen because of headache; this may underestimate the headache problem, because there may be patients with troublesome headaches who, for whatever reason, cannot or do not seek medical advice. Statistics for the United Kingdom tend to minimize this distortion because of the free medical service in Britain. The Morbidity Statistics for General Practice, second national study (1970 to 1971) (3) indicates that in an arbitrarily defined population base of 100,000 residents, in the areas surveyed, 4,000 people between the ages of 25 and 45 went to their general practitioners with a chief

Management of Migraine in the Elderly

complaint of headache; and 1,560 over the age of 65 visited their physician with headache. Again, the inference is that headaches are not rare in the elderly. Furthermore, in this study, the majority of headaches were diagnosed by the general practitioners as either migraine or tension headaches, both in the younger and older age groups.

The elderly with migraine and tension headaches consist of a majority group who have carried their headaches into old age and a smaller group who, some time after the age of 50, developed these headaches de novo. Selby and Lance (4), in their survey of 500 patients attending a migraine clinic, determined that 12 patients (2.4%) began to have migraine between the ages of 50 and 60. Similarly, Lance, Curran, and Anthony (5) reported that 10% of their tension-headache population began to have their headaches after the age of 50.

Epidemiologic studies on cluster headache are fewer, because this entity is uncommon. While cluster headache tends to begin at a somewhat older age than migraine and tension headaches (mean age of onset in a number of series, 31.5 years) (6), they too attenuate with age. However, cluster headache can begin for the first time after the age of 70 (7).

The common functional headaches—tension headache, migraine headaches, and cluster headache—still are very much at the top of the differential diagnosis of headaches in the elderly. Sometimes, they are more difficult to diagnose: first, because they occur in the underbrush of suspicion of the ominous lesions that accompany aging, and second, because these benign functional-headache syndromes, particularly migraine, may change their presentation as the patient ages. For example, some patients who have had typical attacks of classic migraine, with auras followed by headaches, may in later life lose their headaches and have only recurrent painless auras (8). These recurrent focal neurological disturbances may be recognized for what they are, *transient migrainous accompaniments* (TMAs) (9), or may be mistaken for more threatening occurrences. This is especially likely to occur when TMAs begin for the first time after the age of 50, with no prior history of any type of migraine. Some elderly patients, in contrast, lose their auras and continue to have the headaches alone; this sequence of events is less confusing, but still is capable of causing concern if there is a hiatus of months or years between the disappearance of the classic and the advent of the common migraine. In dealing with this problem, Wilkinson offers the prudent advice that "if . . . there is any major change in the location or duration or if there are any focal symptoms or signs present, the possibility of some intracranial pathology such as an intracranial tumor must be considered and the patient fully investigated" (8). To this advice should be added the admonition that various metabolic and biochemical disturbances are equally capable of causing headaches in the elderly, some of which may be confused with migraine or tension headaches. Compounding the problem is that some of these "organic" conditions may exacerbate underlying migraine, making treatment of the migraine difficult or impossible until the underlying condition is identified and resolved.

Cervical spondylosis has been termed "a common and important cause of headache beginning in middle life or later" (10). There is considerable doubt about this, however (11). Most people over the age of 50 have radiologic changes indicating some degree of cervical spondylosis, but few have symptoms (12). The headaches that usually are attributed to cervical spondylosis are dull and of long duration, affect mainly the occiput, are nonpulsatile, and are not aggravated by maneuvers that increase pulse rate or pulse pressure; therefore, they should not be susceptible to confusion with migraine. They do resemble tension headaches—and, indeed, may well be tension headaches.

Vascular hypertension is common in the elderly and is widely believed, by lay people, to be responsible for headaches. In fact, the prevalence of headache is no higher in patients with mild or moderate hypertension than it is in age-matched normotensive populations; it is only in patients with severe chronic hypertension, defined as a diastolic pressure above 130, that headache is distinctly more common (13). These hypertensive headaches are a dull throbbing ache, often more pronounced in the occiput, that wakes the patient early in the monring and is aggravated by bending and straining. The headache clears after the patient has been

TABLE 1 Lesions Producing Headache in the Elderly

Structural
    Cervical spine disease (spondylosis, rheumatoid arthritis)
    Hypertension
    Giant-cell arteritis
    Increased intracranial pressure (subdural hematoma, neoplasm, hydrocephalus)
    Atherothrombotic cerebrovascular disease
    Intracranial hemorrhage
    Meningitis
Metabolic
    Medications
    Respiratory disease (chronic obstructive lung disease, sleep apnea)
    Anemia and polycythemia
    Hypercalcemia
    Renal disease

---

up and about for an hour or so and disappears once the hypertension has been treated successfully. Hypertensive headaches may bear a superficial resemblance to common migraine, but the daily or nearly daily occurrence, the matitudinal timing, and—above all—the finding of high blood pressure, allow differentiation. Sometimes, hypertension may occur in people who already have migraine, and this is a significant juxtaposition for four reasons:

1. Treatment given for the migraine may be causing the hypertension (e.g., ergotamine).
2. Treatment contemplated for the migraine may be contraindicated by the hypertension (e.g., methysergide, ergotamine).
3. Treatment contemplated for the hypertension (e.g., methyldopa) may cause headaches, confounding the assessment of the migraine.
4. The presence of hypertension may make migraine unresponsive to treatment until the blood pressure is brought under control. Fortunately, two major categories of

migraine prophylactic medications are capable of lowering blood pressure (beta blockers and calcium-channel blockers), allowing the opportunity to treat the hypertension and the migraine simultaneously with one agent.

Giant-cell arteritis may produce headaches that can be confused with migraine. It is a rare disease, but becomes less so in an aging population. The incidence of giant-cell arteritis is 9.3 per hundred thousand population per year. The overall prevalence over the age of 50 is 28.6 per hundred thousand; the prevalence increases with age, so that it is 6.8 per hundred thousand in people in thier 50s, but 73.1 per hundred thousand in people in their 80s (14). Giant-cell arteritis may be present with focal headaches, often temporal, sometimes occipital. It also may be associated with visual disturbances, which sometimes may be episodic (before becoming permanent) (15). Occasionally, the headache and the fluctuating visual loss may bring classic migraine to mind, but this possibility should be dismissed quickly once it is appreciated that the patient is experiencing progressively worsening headaches, often on a background of systemic ill-health (malaise, weight loss, myalgias, arthralgias, subjective febrility, night sweats, jaw claudications, etc.). Since, on occasion, the appearance of giant-cell arteritis can be confusing, it is prudent to obtain an erythrocyte sedimentation rate (ESR) in all patients with headache over the age of 50; normal ESRs are rare enough in giant-cell arteritis that the test is a valid screen.

Atherothrombotic vascular disease may be associated with headache, and this opens up vexatious and confusing controversies about the relationship (if any) between migraine and cerebral ischemia, about the distinction between transient ischemic attacks and isolated migraine auras, and about the significance and validity of the concept of TMAs. Here are the parts of this puzzle:

1. Generalized or hemicranial headaches, usually mild, may occur in approximately 25% of patients with transient ischemic attacks or completed strokes produced by atherosclerotic cerebrovascular disease or cardiogenic emboli. The pathogenesis of these headaches is unknown. The classic explanation of headaches being caused by dilation

Management of Migraine in the Elderly

of pain-sensitive collateral circulation (the Willis hypothesis) probably is inaccurate. It may be that the platelets, which are the common factor in atherothrombotic occlusion and embolism to the brain, may in addition to aggregating, lyse, liberating as a result of the "platelet release reaction" vasoactive amines which act downstream on the blood vessel to produce dilation, sterile inflammation, and vascular headaches (16).
2. About 11% of patients with these headaches of ischemic cerebrovascular disease have a previous history of long-term throbbing headaches (17), likely migrainous, thus leading to confusion of the present headaches with migraine.
3. One school of thought about the pathophysiology of migraine holds that platelets are paramount in the production of migraine at all ages; that microembolism of platelets in a patient genetically susceptible to developing the neurophysiologic phenomenon of spreading depression could precipitate this phenomenon, creating symptoms that would be recognized as classic migraine; and that microembolization in a patient not so susceptible would produce either nothing or, depending on the size of the embolus and perhaps on the age of the patient, a transient ischemic attack (18).
4. Some patients with symptoms resembling transient ischemic attacks have, on investigation, no evident cause for them. C. Miller Fisher (9) has raised the possibility that these symptoms may be TMAs—i.e., aura symptoms—detached from headaches. Sometimes these can occur in people with a past history of common or classic migraine; sometimes they arise de novo, often after the age of 50. Fisher has given the following main criteria for the diagnosis of "late-life migrainous accompaniments":
    a. Scintillations or other visual display in the spell; next in order, paresthesias, aphasia, dysarthria, and paralysis
    b. Buildup of scintillations
    c. March of paresthesias (from one body part to the other)

d. Progression from one accompaniment to another, often with a delay
e. The occurrence of two or more similar spells (this helps to exclude embolism)
f. Headache in the spell
g. Episodes that last 15 to 25 minutes
h. Characteristic midlife "flurry"
i. A generally benign course
j. Normal angiography
k. Exlusion of clotting diastheses

To these criteria should be added "establishing that cardiac rhythm and structure are normal," since cardiogenic embolism is a very much underestimated cause of transient ischemic attacks (TIAs) and stroke. The essential trap in the concept of TMAs is that this diagnosis may encourage insufficient investigation of a middle-aged or elderly patient with transient neurological events, leading to the possibility that TIAs (and the accompanying opportunity to prevent stroke) may be missed.

How can we put the pieces of this puzzle together? The safe way is to say that typical presentations of classic or common migraine or of TIAs are not difficult to recognize and should be treated as such, but that atypical headaches (that is, new headaches or different headaches), or the appearance of focal neurological symptoms that are not typical of migraine auras, warrant the closest scrutiny in both the clinic and the laboratory. This scrutiny should include a search for a family history of vascular disease, a search for the presence of stroke-risk factors (hypertension, smoking, diabetes mellitus, hyperlipidemia, or heart disease), and a thorough examination to seek out orbital and cervical bruits, hypertension, unequal blood pressures in the two arms, cardiac arrhythmias, heart murmurs, ventricular hypertrophy, abdominal bruits, peripheral vascular disease, and xanthoma. If any of the foregoing are abnormal, laboratory investigations should be done, including computerized tomography of the brain, electrocardiography (EKG), echocardiography, Doppler studies of the carotid

Management of Migraine in the Elderly

and vertebral arteries, and, if indicated, cerebral angiography. The philosophy behind this recommendation is that it is too easy to write off TIAs as manifestations of migraine and, before a diagnosis of atypical migraine is made in someone over the age of 50, adequate laboratory investigation must be done.

The other structural lesions noted in Table 1 all cause, and indeed may accompany, headache in the elderly, but these headaches are very unlikely to be mistaken for migraine and will not be discussed in detail here.

The metabolic lesions noted in Table 1 are an important consideration in any discussion of migraine in the elderly, because the headaches that these biochemical lesions may produce often are due to vasodilatation and, therefore, are quite susceptible to confusion with migraine.

Medications (see Table 2) can be an important cause of headaches in the elderly; as people age, they develop more diseases and the need for more medications. Some of these medications have headaches as a side effect. Some of these headaches clearly are produced by vasodilation (e.g., nitrates, nicotinic acid, etc.,); in others the pathogenesis of the headache is unclear. The headaches produced by medication are usually diffuse, seldom very severe, sometimes throbbing, and of variable duration. Superficially, they may resemble migraine, but a carefully taken history usually will establish that they are not. A more difficult diagnostic situation exists when medication, rather than producing headache "on its own," triggers underlying migraine. It should be noted that alcohol and caffeine (coffee, tea, and cola drinks) also are pharmacologically active and can cause headache. Any inquiry about medication also should include detailed questions about caffeine and alcohol intake. A good rule is that if a patient on multiple medications develops headaches, any medication that is not absolutely required should be stopped. A sad fact of current medical practice is that this sometimes means that some or all of the medications can be eliminated.

Respiratory disease increases in the elderly, and with it the occurrence of hypercapnia and/or hypoxia. Both may increase cerebral blood flow; provoke intracranial vasodilation; and cause

TABLE 2 An Incomplete List of Medications Producing Headache in the Elderly

Disease	Medication
Cardiovascular	Vasodilators (nitroglycerin, isosorbide dinitrate, nylidrin, nicotinic acid, dipyridamole)
	Hypotensives (methyldopa, reserpine, etc.,)
	Antiarrhythmics (quinidine, disopyramide, digoxin)
Respiratory	Bronchodilators (theophylline, pseudoephedrine, etc.)
Musculoskeletal	NSAIDs (e.g., indomethacin), carisoprodal
Gastrointestinal	H_2 blockers (ranitidine)
Central nervous system	Sedatives (benzodiazepines, barbiturates, alcohol)
	Stimulants (caffeine, methylphenidate, pemoline)
	Antiparkinson (l-dopa, amantadine)
Gynecological	Supplemental estrogens
Infectious	Trimethoprim-sulfamethoxazole antibiotics
Oncologic	Chemotherapeutics (tamoxifen, diethylstilbestrol, cyclophosphamide)

dull, diffuse, and often throbbing headaches, which may come on at any time but frequently are worse in the morning. Chronic obstructive lung disease (e.g., emphysema) is particularly likely to do this. The headaches produced by chronic obstructive lung disease can be compounded, because some of the bronchodilator medications prescribed for this condition (e.g., theophylline) themselves can produce headache. Furthermore, many people with chronic respiratory disease develop a degree of secondary polycythemia, with increased blood volume and consequent intracranial vasodilation, sometimes with increased intracranial pressure; not infrequently, polycythemia either presents with or is accompanied by headache. Sleep apnea is a common problem in the elderly, particularly the obese elderly with lax upper airway tissues and a degree of underlying chronic pulmonary disease. Persons with sleep apnea frequently awaken in a groggy, headachey state, with their head clearing sometime after they get up and about.

A similar groggy, headachy state may result from *hypercalcemia*. In the elderly, hypercalcemia usually represents underlying malignancy, such as carcinoma of the prostate with bony metastases. *Chronic renal disease* also may product headache, for reasons that are presently obscure. Severe degrees of *anemia* may, through the agency of increased cerebral blood flow and intracranial vasodilation, produce a throbbing holocephalic headache; headache in anemia is not likely to occur unless the hemoglobin content is reduced by at least 50%.

In summary, the elderly are subject to a great array of structural and metabolic lesions that can produce headache, and some of these headaches may mimic migraine. These facts highlight the need for extra care in dealing with the elderly headache patient, the importance of a high index of suspicion, and the wisdom of investigating thoroughly any headache pattern that is the least bit atypical.

PROBLEMS OF TREATING MIGRAINE IN THE ELDERLY

As we age, we accumulate illnesses. At times, these illnesses may contraindicate medication that otherwise might be prescribed for the treatment of migraine. Table 3 is a partial compilation of those diseases that are not particularly uncommon in the elderly and of the various migraine medications that they bar.

An equally serious problem of treating migraine in the elderly is that older people, with their reserves diminished by the physiologic changes of age and by intercurrent illness, may be more likely than younger people to develop side effects to antimigraine medication. At times, it is difficult to know whether the medication is unmasking occult coexistent disease or producing symptoms de novo. For example, older people are much more likely to become sedated and confused with the doses of tricyclic antidepressants that are customarily used to prevent attacks of migraine.

TABLE 3 Contraindications to Antimigraine Medications in the Elderly

Antimigraine Medication	May cause or aggravate
Analgesics	
ASA	Peptic ulcer
Acetaminophen	Renal disease, liver disease
Codeine	Constipation
Barbiturates	Mental slowing and confusion
Ergotamine and dihydroergotamine	Hypertension, peripheral athersclerotic vascular disease, Raynaud's diseae, coronary heart disease, cerebrovascular disease
Prophylactics	
Tricyclics	Glaucoma, prostatism, cardiac arrhythmias, sedation
Beta blockers	Heart block, bronchospasm, hypotension, heart failure, depression
Calcium blockers	Heart block, heart failure, peripheral edema, hypotension, constipation
Methysergide	Retroperitoneal and pleuropulmonary fibrosis, peripheral vascular disease, renal disease, ischemic cardiac disease, cardiac valvular disease

Do these symptoms occur because the anticholinergic effects of the tricyclic are unmasking an underlying defect in cholinergic neurotransmission in a patient with heretofore silent (subclinical) Alzheimer's disease? Or are these anticholinergic effects overwhelming cholinergic neurotransmission in a previously healthy neuronal system, free of disease, but depleted by the normal neuronal and neurotransmitter dropout that attends normal old age? The answer is as yet unknown and, in any event, academic. The practical point is that the tricyclic antidepressants may be used when there are no contraindications (see Table 3), but when

Management of Migraine in the Elderly

used, they should be started in very small dosages (e.g., 10 mg per day) and increased in very small steps (e.g., by 10 mg every four days) until an appropriate maintenance dosage is reached.

Similarly, the barbiturates that are incorporated into some analgesic-sedative compounds may have no adverse effects (other than the risk of addiction) in the younger individual, but in an older patient they may produce, especially if taken frequently, depression, confusion, and sometimes paradoxical excitement. The use of barbiturates is justifiably on the decline because of their relatively low therapeutic index, the problems with tolerance, the liability for abuse, and the number of drug interactions (19); it is reasonable, therefore, to recommend that no formulation containing barbiturates be used for the treatment of migraine in the elderly.

The use of ergotamine and its congeners (e.g., methysergide) creates equal problems in the elderly. These drugs have vasoconstriction properties that are capable of producing signs and symptoms of vascular insufficiency involving the limbs, eyes, heart, and brain (20). In younger people with normal vascular systems, these symptoms rarely occur. In older people, where there is preexistent vascular disease (often asymptomatic), the administration of these ergot derivatives easily may provoke symptoms and signs of vascular insufficiency, often with most unfortunate consequences. Accordingly, it is reasonable to recommend that ergot derivatives not be given to people over the age of 60.

In summary, the prevalence of incidental illness and the increased susceptibility to the development of side effects from medication in the elderly pose problems in the treatment of migraine. These problems can be minimized by:

1. Always knowing the general condition of the elderly person thoroughly before prescribing medication
2. Prescribing medication in very small initial dosages
3. Increasing the dosage of medication very slowly, keeping the patient under close clinical and laboratory follow-up

SUMMARY

Migraine is not uncommon in the elderly. Rarely, it may begin after the age of 60; more often, it is carried over from youth and middle age. As the migraine is carried over, however, it may change its pattern, producing some diagnostic confusion with diseases peculiar to the aged, particularly cerebrovascular disease. Careful attention to history, meticulous examination, and appropriate investigations usually will permit differentiation between atypical migraine and cerebrovascular insufficiency. As older patients develop still more incidental illnesses (for example, respiratory disease with hypercapnia and hypoxia), they may develop headache as manifestations of these diseases; these headaches, too, can be diagnosed by a careful clinician who is aware of all the possibilities. Many of these incidental diseases call for medication, and many of these medications themselves can cause headache. The problem of medication-induced headache is best addressed by being alert to the possibility; by carefully assessing, in a hard-nosed fashion, the need for each medication that the patient takes; and by ruthlessly eliminating all unnecessary medications.

The treatment of migraine is made difficult in the elderly by the increased burden of incidental illness in this older age group, which usually poses significant contraindications to some of the medications used to treat migraine. The problem is compounded further by the fact that the elderly are particularly susceptible to developing side effects to medications. These problems with medications, however, usually can be overcome by being very familiar with the older patient's general medical condition, by keeping the medications prescribed for migraine to a minimum, by starting those medications in a small dosage and increasing it gradually, and by keeping the patient under careful clinical and laboratory supervision.

The management of migraine in the elderly is a challenge, but one that usually can be met by the thorough and prudent physician. Nothing good ever came easily.

REFERENCES

1. Whitty, C. W. M. and Hockaday, J. (1968). Migraine, a follow-up study of 92 patients, *Brit. Med. J. 1*: 735-736.
2. Waters, W. E. (1974). The Pontypridd headache survery, *Headache, 14*: 81-90.
3. Royal College of Practitioners, Office of Population Consensus and Surveys, and Department of Health and Social Security (1974). Morbidity statistics from general practice: Second national study 1970-71, studies on medical and population subjects No. 26, Her Magesty's Stationery Office, London.
4. Selby, G. and Lance, J. W. (1960). Observations on 500 cases of migraine and allied vascular headache, *J. Neurol. Neurosurg. Psychiat., 23*: 23-32.
5. Lance, J. W., Curran, D. A., and Anthony, M. (1965). Investigations into the mechanism and treatment of chronic headache, *Med. J. Austral., 2*: 909-912.
6. Sjaastad, O. (1986). Cluster headache, *Handbook of Clinical Neurology* vol. 4(48), (P. J. Vinken, G. W. Bruyn, H. Klawans, and F. C. Rose, eds.) Elsevier Science Publishers, Amsterdam, pp. 217-246.
7. Sutherland, J. M. and Eadie M. J. (1972). Cluster headache, *Research and Clinical Studies in Headache*, Vol. 3 (A. P. Friedman, ed.) Karger, Basel, pp. 92-125.
8. Wilkinson, M. (1986). Clincial features of migraine, *Handbook of Clinical Neurology*, Vol. 4(48) (P. J. Vinken, G. W. Bruyn, H. Klawans, and F. C. Rose, eds.) Elsevier Science Publishers, Amsterdam, pp. 117-133.
9. Fisher, C. M. (1980). Late-life migraine accompaniments as a cause of unexplained transient ischemic attacks, *Can. J. Neurol. Sci., 7*: 9-18.
10. Brain, W. R. Some unresolved problems of cervical spondylosis, *Brit. Med. J., 1*: 771-777.
11. Edmeads, J. (1978). Headaches with diseases of the cervical spine, *Med. Clin. N. Amer., 62*: 533-544.
12. Elias, F.. (1958). Roentgen findings in the asymptomatic cervical spine, *NY State J. Med., 58*: 3300-3303.
13. Badran, R. H., Weir, R. J., and McGuinness, J. B. (1970). Hypertension and headache, *Scott Med. J., 15*: 48-51.

14. Bengtsson, B. A. (1982). Incidence of giant cell arteritis, *Acta Med. Scand. Suppl., 658*: 15-17.
15. Ross Russell, R. W. (1986). Giant cell (cranial) arteritis, *Handbook of Clinical Neurology*, Vol. 4(48) (P. J. Vinken, G. W. Bruyn, H. Klawans, and F. C. Rose, eds.), Elsevier Science Publishers, Amsterdam, pp. 309-328.
16. Edmeads, J. (1979). The headache of ischemic cerebrovascular disease, *Headache, 19*: 345-349.
17. Portenoy, R. K., Abissi, C. J., Lipton, R. B., et al. (1984). Headache in cerebrovascular disease, *Stroke, 15*: 1009-1012.
18. Peatfield, R. C. (1987). Can transient ischemic attacks and classical migraine always be distinguished? *Headache, 27*: 240-243.
19. Harvey, S. C. (1985). Hypnotics and sedatives, Goodman and Gilman's *Pharmacological Basis of Therapeutics*, 7th ed. (A. G. Gilman, L. S. Goodman, T. W. Rall, and F. Murad, eds.), Macmillan, New York, pp. 339-371.
20. Senter, J. H., Liberman, A. N., and Pinte, R. Cerebral manifestations of ergotism. Report on a case and review of the literature, *Stroke, 7*: 88-92.

9

Migraine in Childhood

A. David Rothner *Cleveland Clinic Foundation, Cleveland, Ohio*

INTRODUCTION

Headache is a common disorder, in children and in adults (1), and results in significant discomfort, as well as time lost from school and work. Often, it also alters the lifestyles of both children and adults. Both physical and psychological etiologies must be investigated to arrive at the correct diagnosis and begin proper treatment. Deciding whther a child's headache is organic or functional is difficult. A thorough and systematic history and examination, coupled with selected laboratory tests, usually will guide the practitioner to the correct diagnosis. The history, epidemiology, etiology, evaluation, and treatment of migraine headaches in children are reviewed in this chapter.

HISTORY

Although historical references to headache date back to 3000 B.C.E., when Sumerian and Babylonian references have been noted, it was not until 460 B.C.E. that Hippocrates described migraine. The term *hemicrania* was coined by Galen (131-201 C.E.). Additional references to migraine in art, music, and literature have been reviewed by Friedman (2). Interestingly, none of the aforementioned references specifically mentions children having this common form of headache. In 1873, Willian Henry Day, a British pediatrician, devoted a chapter of his book, *Essays on Diseases of Children* (3), to the subject of headache in children. Although he described primarily nonvascular headaches and felt that they were due to "bad arrangement" in the lives of children, he also referred to vascular headaches. A major milestone in the study of pediatric headaches occurred in 1962, when Bille (4) reported on a study of 9,000 schoolchildren in Sweden, with specific references to the various types of headaches noted. To date, only three books devoted entirely to the subject of headache in children have been published (5-7).

It is of interest that Lewis Carroll, author of the much-loved *Alice in Wonderland*, suffered from migraine; his migrainous hallucinations served as the imagery for Alice's changes in size.

EPIDEMIOLOGY

Headache surveys generate varying results, depending on whether an entire community is surveyed or the study is composed of people who visit a general physician's office or a specialist's office. In the former case, headache sufferers who do not seek medical attention are surveyed; in the latter instance, patients who do seek medical attention receive the study's attention. However, some generalities can be made.

The prevalence of all types of headache increases with age until approximately age 50, when headache frequency begins to diminish. In the monumental study by Bille (4), where an entire population of children was studied, it was noted that by age 7, 2.5% of the children had frequent nonmigrainous headache, 1.4% had true migraine, and 35% had infrequent headaches of other varieties. By age 15, 15.7% had frequent nonmigrainous headaches, 5.3% had migraine, and 54% had infrequent headaches of other varieties. The frequency of headache in prepubertal males is higher than in prepubertal females; once puberty has been reached, the frequency of all types of headaches in women is higher. Jay and Tomasi (8) noted that headache accounted for 22% of all new patient diagnoses in a pediatric neurology outpatient clinic. Our statistics at the Cleveland Clinic Foundation confirm this percentage, and other studies (9) have substantiated these figures.

CLASSIFICATION AND ETIOLOGY

There is no single, agreed-upon definition of headache or classification of headaches in adults. The classifications most commonly referred to are those of the Ad Hoc Committee on Classification of Headache, published in 1962 (10), and of the World Federation of Neurology, published by the Migraine and Headache Research Group in 1973 (11). The classification of headaches currently is being reviewed by the International Headache Society. In addition to the above definitions, I find it useful to classify headaches based on their temporal pattern; i.e., acute headaches, acute recurrent headaches (migraine), chronic progressive headaches (organic), and chronic nonprogressive headaches (psychogenic) (12). Migraine headaches are classified further to include classic migraine; common migraine; complicated migraine; including ophthalmoplegic and hemiplegic migraine; and migraine variants—including confusional migraine, benign paroxysmal vertigo, paroxysmal torticollis, basilar artery migraine, the periodic syndrome, and migraine precipitated by head trauma (13).

THE EVALUATION

To properly diagnose and effectively treat a patient with headaches, the physician must understand the basic pathophysiology and mechanism of the headaches, as well as the clinical and emotional aspects of the problem. The vast majority of headaches can be diagnosed correctly by a thorough, detailed, and well-organized history. This is the key to correct diagnosis and mandatory to differentiate one headache type from another. The questions should be directed to both the parents and the child. One frequently is surprised by the amount of information a young child can volunteer. In adolescents, a private interview may be helpful. The answers to specific questions are needed to generate sufficient data upon which to base the diagnosis (see Table 1).

When dealing with children data also must include information regarding pregnancy, labor, and delivery; growth and development; behavior; academic functions; family history; and the presence or absence of previous encephalopathic events. A systematic review must look specifically at medical conditions that may contribute

TABLE 1 Headache Data Base

1. Do you have a single type of headache or several types?
2. When did the headache start?
3. How did the headache start (trauma, life event)?
4. How often does the headache occur?
5. Is the headache becoming more severe?
6. Is the headache occurring more frequently?
7. Is there anything that provokes a headache (food, activity, situation)?
8. Can you tell that a headache is about to start (warning)?
9. Where is the pain located?
10. What does the pain feel like?
11. What other symptoms do you have when the headache is present (nausea, vomiting, dizziness, etc.)?
12. Do you stop what you are normally doing when you have the headache?
13. How long does the headache last?
14. What makes the headache better?
15. Do you have any other medical problems (asthma, allergies)?
16. Are you taking any medications regularly?
17. Does anyone else in your family have bad headaches?
18. Has anything particularly good or bad happened in your personal life or in your family life recently (death, divorce, graduation)?
19. What do you think is causing your headaches?
20. What do you think helps make them better?

Migraine in Childhood

to the patient's headache problem, as well as the use of medications that may precipitate or provoke headaches and those used to treat headaches. An additional set of questions must deal with the presence or absence of symptoms of increased intracranial pressure (IICP), including nausea, vomiting, ataxia, focal weakness, visual problems, seizures, personality change, and lethargy. If symptoms of either IICP or loss of previously acquired neurological milestones (regression) are present, an organic process is suspected and the evaluation must be accelerated. Throughout the examination, it is important to note the affect of the child and the parents, as well as their interaction. Specific symptoms—such as the onset of severe headache without previously noted headache, persistently localized headache, headache associated with neurologic symptoms or signs, headache associated with straining, a change in a previous headache pattern, or pain that awakens a child from sleep—also suggest an organic disorder. At the conclusion of the history, one should have an initial impression of the headache type, the presence or absence of IICP, and the presence or absence of a progressive neurological disorder.

The general physical examination is normal in the majority of patients with muscle-contraction headaches or migraine headaches. However, contributing etiologies can be noted on the general examination. The measurement of blood pressure with varying sized cuffs in children is mandatory, as is seeking cutaneous markers such as café au lait spots, which can be seen in neurofibromatosis and may lead to a diagnosis of vascular disease, CNS neoplasm, or hydrocephalus. The neurologic examination in children determines the integrity of the central nervous system and is expanded to include measurement of the cranial circumference and auscultation of the cranium for bruits. If loud, asymmetric, machinery-like murmurs are heard, an arteriovenous malformation should be suspected. Funduscopic examination is difficult in children and often is best postponed until the end of the examination, so as not to lose the cooperation of the child. The pediatric neurologic examination is discussed elsewhere (14).

The choice of laboratory tests depends on the differential diagnosis. Foremost considerations are space-occupying lesions, seizures, and other paroxysmal nonepileptiform disorders. In most patients, roentgenograms of the skull are not necessary. The EEG is of limited value in the routine evaluation of headache. Nonspecific abnormalities are noted frequently, especially in children, and are not significant. Epileptiform discharges are seen with an increased frequency in children with migraine who do not have any seizure disorder (15). Both CT and MRI are safe, accurate, and rapid methods of evaluating the intracranial contents. Both types of scans are useful in a wide variety of conditions and in evaluating headaches that may be organic in etiology. If a patient has progressive symptomatology—symptoms of IICP or focal symptomatology—if the neurologic examination shows any abnormality, if neurocutaneous stigmata or macrocephaly are present, or if any laboratory test such as an EEG points to a focal lesion, an imaging procedure is mandatory to rule out a structural abnormality. The imaging study should include the paranasal sinuses. Further invasive studies, such as arteriography, pneumoencephalography, and PET, all may be useful under special circumstances, but are not used routinely in the evaluation of headache patients. On rare occasions, a lumbar puncture is useful in determining the presence of an infectious process or in measuring the CSF pressure in pseudotumor cerebri after a space-occupying lesion has been ruled out. Sedation may be necessary. In other patients who have emotional problems associated with their headache, or if home/school difficulties seem to be playing a role, tests of general intellectual function may be useful, as may be projective testing or an interview with a psychologist or psychiatrist.

PATHOPHYSIOLOGY

There is no reason to suspect that the etiopathogenesis of the migraine attack in children is any different from that of the migraine attack in adults. The basic etiopathogenesis still is not fully understood. In 1873, Liveing (16) suggested that migraine was similar to epilepsy and that circulatory changes were secondary to CNS discharges. In the ensuing hundred years, a vascular theory promulgated by Graham and Wolff (17) became popular, and further information was gathered concerning blood-flow studies in migraine, as well as the role of neurotransmitters (18). Currently, we have returned to the initial theory that vascular changes in the migraine attack probably are initiated in the central nervous system (19). Further elucidation of the etiology and pathophysiology of this disorder is necessary to arrive at more definitive therapy.

An acute headache is defined as a single event without a history of similar events. The most likely etiology is an acute illness. This subject has been reviewed by Kandt and Levine (20). Acute and recurrent headaches usually are migraine and will be discussed later in this chapter. Chronic and progressive headaches usually are due to IICP and increase both in severity and frequency over time (21). Chronic nonprogressive headaches occur daily, or multiple times weekly, and are relatively consistent, without significant change in severity, without symptoms of IICP, and without neurologic signs. Chronic nonprogressive headaches usually are functional in origin. The subject has not been well studied in pediatric and adolescent patients, and a better understanding of this form of headache is needed (22).

THE MIGRAINE SYNDROME

The World Federation of Neurology defines migraine as "a familial disorder characterized by recurrent attacks of headache, widely variable in intensity, frequency, and duration. Attacks are commonly unilateral and are usually associated with anorexia, nausea, and vomiting. In some cases, they are associated with neurological and mood disturbances (11). Prensky and Sommer (23) have described criteria for the diagnosis of childhood migraine. These authors suggest that to diagnose migraine properly, patients with recurrent headaches separated by symptom-free intervals should have three of the following six symptoms: (a) abdominal pain, nausea, or vomiting with the headache; (b) hemicrania; (c) throbbing pulsatile pain; (d) complete relief after a brief period of rest; (e) an aura, either visual, sensory, or motor; and (f) a history of migraine headaches in one or more members of the immediate family. I feel that these criteria are useful, but need further explanation. Since common migraine is more frequent than classic migraine in children, it is obvious that hemicrania is seen less commonly than are bifrontal or bitemporal headaches, so that hemicrania is not necessarily an absolute requirement. In addition, since classic migraine is less common than common migraine, an aura rarely is seen in pediatrics unless it is autonomic in nature. The relief seen after a brief period of sleep frequently is incomplete in children, although sleep is beneficial. In our group of patients, the usual symptoms associated with an attack of migraine included nausea and vomiting, abdominal pain (90%), relief after sleep (90%), a positive family history (69%), a throbbing quality (58%), a unilateral headache (36%), and an aura (17%) (13).

THE MIGRAINE SUBSTRATE

Migraine attacks often are precipitated by trigger phenomena. Studying these triggers has been difficult, and adequate documentation of their role in the pathogenesis of migraine is not available. Provocative factors that have been mentioned frequently include anxiety, stress, fatigue, excessive sleep, minor head injury, exercise, menses, travel, illness, diet, odors, medications, and hunger. Specific foods have been implicated on numerous occasions and, although allergies to these foods have been discussed, the more commonly held belief is that the vasoactive substances in these foods initiate a vascular reaction. The most common foods implicated inlude preserved meats such as bacon, ham, and salami, due to the presence of nitrate; aged cheese and red wine, due to the presence of tyramine; oriental food, due to MSG; and chocolate, due to phenylethylamine. Proof that these chemicals actually precipitate migraine is not conclusive. Other researchers have claimed that the use of an allogoantigenic has been useful, especially in refractory patients (24).

Disagreement as to whether or not a true migraine personality exists has persisted over the years. Some researchers have suggested that migraine attacks are precipitated by pernicious emotional reactions. Others state that children with migraine are shy,

Migraine in Childhood

withdrawn, extremely obedient, stubborn, and inflexible (25). Bille (4) added to this description by stating that migrainous children are fearful, tense, sensitive, and easily frustrated. However, he concluded that there was no demonstrable difference in social class, intelligence, ambition, or nervous symptoms in patients with migraine. Additional studies (25,26) performed more recently using standard personality inventories have not demonstrated that there is a migrainous personality or that the personalities of migraineurs deviate from those of the general population. It should be noted that patients who are more bothered by their pain may indeed seek more help and have the aforementioned traits.

Most authors feel that migraine is a hereditary disorder, although some disagreement exists regarding the mode of inheritance (27). There is no question that there is an increased frequency of this disorder in families. Interestingly, when one looks at the parents and siblings of migrainous patients, 46% have a positive family history, compared to 18% of patients with tension headaches. If grandparents are included, 55% of patients have a positive family history. In our own studies, 65% of patients had a positive family history; in the cumulative series published by Prensky (23), 44% to 85% of patients had a positive family history. Whether the disorder is inherited as an autosomal dominant with variable penetrance or is a complex and multifactorial hereditary disorder has not yet been determined.

A number of interesting correlations that have been made regarding pediatric migraine should be emphasized. These include an increased incidence of car sickness, sleep disturbances, syncope, mitral valve prolapse, and Tourette syndrome (28–30).

There are some differences between pediatric and adult migraine (31). Common migraine is more frequent in children than in adults. In children, therefore, there is a decreased frequency of visual aura and of hemicrania. In addition, children may be less able to describe the aura seen in classic migraine. Also, children appear to have fewer attacks per month. Their attacks tend to occur late in the day, rather than early in the morning. The attacks tend to be shorter in duration. Attacks in children tend to be relieved by sleep, and their headaches seem to be more easily controlled.

As children mature into adolescents, further changes occur in the pattern of migrainous attacks. These include an increased frequency of classic migraine as opposed to common migraine, an increased frequency of hemicrania, an increased frequency in the number of attacks per month, a tendency for the attacks to occur in the morning as opposed to the afternoon, an increased duration of attacks, and an increased difficulty in bringing the attacks under control. In addition, during later adolescence, mixed-headache pattern begins to emerge; i.e., severe paroxysmal headaches with nausea or vomiting several times per month are superimposed on a pattern of daily headaches (32).

TYPES OF MIGRAINE

Classic migraine occurs less frequently in children and adolescents than in adults and is less frequent than common migraine in children. It occurred in approximately 15% of the patients in our series (15). Classic migraine is preceded by a visual aura—most commonly, blurred vision. Other manifestations include brightly colored lights, moving lights, distorted images, scotomata, and fortification spectra. Differences in somatic perceptions known as the *Alice in Wonderland syndrome* also may occur. Somatic disturbances—including dysphasia, dysesthesia, hemiplegia, and speech disturbances—are less frequent. The auras in children have not been well studied, but usually last 20 minutes. The headache is contralateral to the aura; is described as orbital, retro-orbital, or frontal; and often is described as severe and throbbing. Abdominal pain, nausea, and vomiting may occur. At this time, children frequently will retire to their rooms. They prefer the room to be dark and quiet and attempt to sleep, knowing that sleep frequently relieves their pain. In our study, attacks occurred one to two times per month and lasted two to six hours. As children mature into adolescents, the attacks grow longer and more frequent and become more difficult to treat (Figure 1).

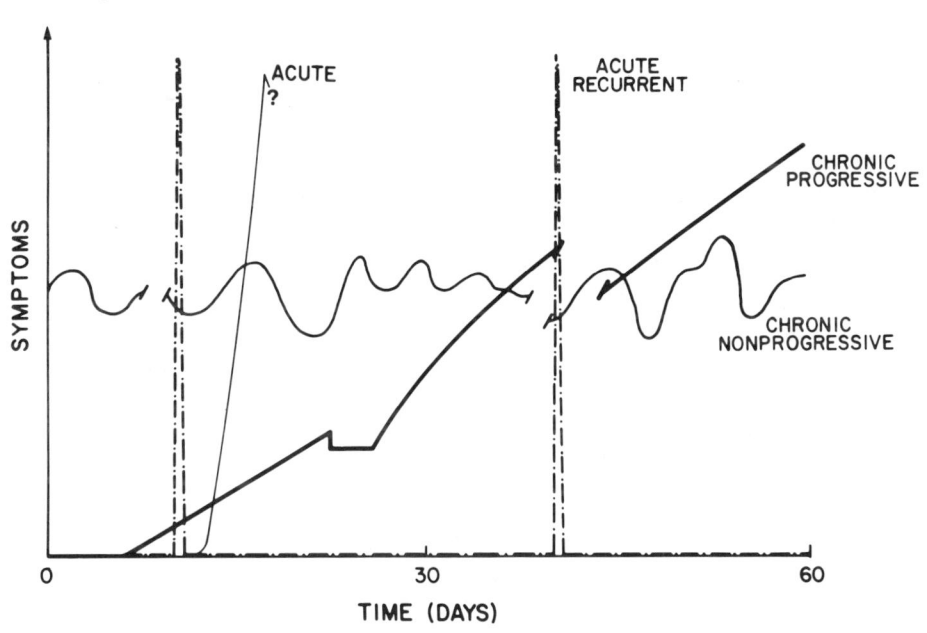

FIGURE 1 Headache types.

Common migraine is the most prevalent form of migraine in children and adolescents and occurred in 70% of our patients. The visual aura common in classic migraine is not present. Instead, an autonomic aura occurs and includes personality change, irritability, and lethargy. Patients are described as pale and having rings under their eyes. This autonomic aura may last anywhere from 30 minutes to several hours and is followed by headache. The headache may be unilateral, but more frequently is bifrontal or generalized. It is described as throbbing and severe. It is followed by anorexia, nausea, vomiting, and abdominal pain. Children frequently prefer a dark, quiet place and attempt to sleep, since their symptoms often are relieved by sleep. Most patients awake feeling refreshed. The entire episode lasts two to six hours and occurs one to two times per month. It seldom is associated with neurologic symptoms or signs.

Complex/complicated migraine is characterized by the association of headache with transient neurologic disturbances. The neurologic deficits are secondary to vasoconstriction, and the syndromes are described by the vascular territories affected and the resultant neurologic symptoms. Most attacks resolve spontaneously but, on occasion, permanent neurologic sequelae occur. When patients with the combination of headache and neurologic signs are seen, it becomes important to differentiate complicated migraine from more serious intracranial conditions such as stroke. The incidence of complicated migraine is not known. Most patients with neurologic correlates of migraine require imaging studies and electroencephalography. It should be noted that angiography during an acute migrainous attack may exacerbate the patient's symptoms (33).

Hemiplegic migraine is the association of recurrent hemiparesis and headache (34). The hemiparesis may precede, accompany, or follow the headache. The headache usually resolves before resolution of the hemiparesis. The headache is contralateral to the hemiparesis. Vasoconstriction, thought to be the etiology, produces ischemia in the distribution of the middle cerebral artery and resultant hemiparesis. If the attacks alternate from side to side, unilateral vascular abnormalities are less likely. To rule out a more serious underlying neurologic disease, patients with hemiplegic migraine should have MRI or enhanced CT scanning. Angiography generally is not required. An aphasia may accompany the hemiparesis if the dominant hemisphere is involved. The differential diagnosis includes thromboembolism, arteriovenous malformation, and tumor. If patients have cardiac disease, are taking oral contraceptives, or have sickle-cell anemia, those disorders may be causative. If the headache is associated with a stiff neck, a lumbar puncture may be indicated to rule out hemorrhage. CSF pleocytosis has been reported to occur during hemiplegic migraine attacks. Mild head trauma may precipitate the attacks. The attacks may be familial.

Ophthalmoplegic migraine is the association of a complete or incomplete third-nerve palsy and ipsilateral headache (35). Once again, the headache may precede, accompany, or follow the

Migraine in Childhood

neurologic abnormality. The pain is retro-orbital and described by patients as severe. The neurological examination is normal, except for a dilated pupil that reacts poorly to light. The eye is deviated laterally because of the unopposed action of the sixth nerve. Patients also may have ptosis and may complain of diplopia. The ophthalmoplegia persists for a variable period of time after the headache has disappeared. Permanent sequelae do occur, but are rare. The third nerve dysfunction is thought to be secondary to edema of the internal carotid area within the cavernous sinus or edema of the distal basilar artery. The differential diagnoses of patients with a painful third-nerve palsy include an aneurysm at the junction of the internal carotid artery and posterior communicating artery, as well as the Tolosa-Hunt syndrome.

Basilar artery migraine was described by Bickerstaff in 1961 (36). It is identified by recurrent attacks of occipital headache in conjunction with neurologic symptomatology referable to the cerebellum and brain stem. This syndrome affects adolescents more frequently than it does adults and occurred in 15% of our series. Because of involvement of the occipital cortices, the patients may present with blurred vision or visual field cuts. They also may have bilateral sensory symptoms, dizziness, vertigo, ataxia, dysarthria, obtundation, quadriparesis, and loss of consciousness. These symptoms may precede the occipital headache. Nausea and vomiting frequently follow the headache. The duration of the attack is several hours, and the symptoms usually clear completely. The differential diagnoses include temporal-lobe epilepsy, vascular disease, demyelinating disease, and occipital neuralgia (37). Electroencephalography between or during attacks may reveal occipital spike discharges. Neurologic evaluation, including imaging study, is recommended.

Acute confusional migraine is a disorder that simulates a toxic encephalopathy (38). The usual scenario is that an adolescent develops a headache that is rapidly followed by confusion and a communicative disorder, including an expressive or receptive aphasia. The patient frequently is referred to the hospital, as drug abuse is suspected. Neurological examination usually does not show focal features, but rather global confusion. The workups of such patients should include toxicology screening, electroencephalography, imaging study, and possible lumbar puncture to rule out encephalitis. The EEG usually shows slowing over the dominant hemisphere (39). The other studies usually are negative. The disorder usually clears within 6 to 12 hours. This syndrome may appear as the first manifestation of migraine or may appear in individuals who have had previous migraine attacks or previous episodes of confusion. The attacks may become recurrent. Nausea and vomiting may occur, but are less prominent. Data concerning the efficacy of preventive measures in such attacks are not available.

MIGRAINE VARIANTS

Migraine variants are defined as episodic, recurrent, transient dysfunctions in a patient who is known to have migraine, a patient who later develops migraine, or a patient who has a family history of migraine. Headache may not be present (40).

Paroxysmal vertigo usually occurs in children between the ages of two and seven (41). The episodes are sudden and brief and involve no alteration of consciousness. Nystagmus may be reported. Headache is not a prominent symptom. Patients fall to the floor and sit in a confused and fearful manner, since they are vertiginous. The attacks usually cease spontaneously within minutes and recur several times per week or several times per month and then disappear spontaneously. If other symptoms and signs of posterior fossa dysfunction are absent, the diagnosis can be made on clinical grounds. If any suspicion of a posterior fossa mass lesion exists, MRI scanning is necessary. The prognosis is generally good. Attacks can be diminished by the use of antihistamines such as diphenydramine. Patients may develop migraine in later years.

Paroxysmal torticollis is a rare, self-limited, benign migraine variant (42). It consists of episodic head tilt variably associated with headaches, nausea, and vomiting. The episodes last from hours to days and clear spontaneously. They recur over several months and then disappear spontaneously. Data concerning the treatment of this disorder are not available.

Alternating hemiplegia is considered by some researchers to be a migraine variant (43). It is a rare disorder that begins in infancy, before the ages of three to five. Patients have recurrent episodes of hemiparesis that frequently alternates sides. Headache is present, but variable in severity. Patients frequently are hypotonic during the episodes, and nausea and vomiting are not part of the picture. Recovery occurs within hours to days, but frequent recurrence is the rule. The episodes seem to be helped by sleep. Angiography does not reveal any vascular abnormalities. Biochemical evaluation for metabolic disorders is negative. If children have numerous hemiplegic attacks, permanent neurologic residua may occur. Treatment with the usual forms of antimigraine therapy have not been successful. Flunarazine, a calcium-channel blocker available in Europe, appears to be helpful.

The periodic syndrome refers to paroxysmal episodes of either abdominal pain or recurrent vomiting in young children, which may lead to dehydration acidosis and recurrent hospitalization (40). Structural abnormalities of the gastrointestinal tract must be ruled out before making this diagnosis. Epilepsy is not usually the cause, especially if no other typical epileptiform attacks occur and there is no loss of consciousness. Clinicians should not be misled by the occasional abnormal EEG that may be noted in such patients. Many patients have a positive family history of migraine. If spells are recurrent, the usual prophylactic forms of antimigraine therapy should be used.

Migraine sine-hemicrania refers to migrainous phenomena such as scintillating scotomata in the absence of headache (44). The disorder should be diagnosed only if the patient has other forms of migraine or has a strong family history of migraine. Other visual phenomena that can occur without headache include monocular scotomata, blindness, and homonymous hemianopia. The attacks are brief, usually lasting for 5 to 30 minutes. Adequate data concerning prophylactic treatment of these phenomena are not available, although some researchers have suggested the chronic use of salicylates.

Patients exhibiting migrainous phenomena following mild head trauma are seen frequently (45). These patients may have neurologic symptomatology ranging from total blindness to hemiplegia, hemisensory phenomenon, severe headache, nausea, and vomiting. The episodes are unique in that the patients have a family history of migraine or a previous migraine history themselves and in that the head injury is insufficient to cause a concussion. The migraine phenomenon, once it occurs, is rather stereotyped. The patient recovers in several hours and there usually are no residua. Once again, adequate data concerning the prophylaxis of these attacks are not available, although some researchers have suggested using propranolol.

Many authors have referred to a syndrome called the *epilepsy-equivalent syndrome*. I think that many of these patients have migraine. Both disorders are common, and epilepsy and migraine may coexist in a single patient. Data concerning the relationship of these two disorders have been presented recently (46). Headaches, nausea, and vomiting, with specific or nonspecific EEG abnormalities, although they may have been diagnosed as seizure equivalents, probably represent migraine. Kinast et al. (15) reported the presence of benign focal epileptiform discharges in 9% of children with migraine, none of whom had epilepsy. Both disorders can present with altered consciousness, abnormal movements, postspell depression, and headache. If the episodes are definitely epileptiform, antiepileptic drugs should be used. Patients who have migraine should not be treated with anticonvulsants.

TREATMENT

The approach to the patient with migraine must be individualized, based on the frequency and severity of the attacks, the presence of an aura, the reliability of the patient, the family's attitude toward the use of medication, and the patient's age (13). Patients with infrequent attacks, once assured and reassured that no underlying neurologic disorder is present, seem to have even less frequent attacks. Nonpharmacologic methods of dealing with migraine—including relaxation therapy, hypnosis, and biofeedback—have gained importance (47). Data have been presented that show that these methodologies can be quite effective. It should be emphasized that biofeedback treatment involves interaction among the patient, the patient's family, and the therapist. Dietary methods to modify the frequency and severity of migraine attacks have been discussed over the years. In approximately 5% to 10% of patients, the families are able to recognize known trigger substances, such as chocolate, preserved meats, or oriental foods (24). In these cases, the substances within the foods are vasoactive and initiate the migraine cascade. The routine use of oligoantigenic diets or elimination diets in migraine patients is not indicated, unless the migraine has been severe and refractory to usual treatment attempts. There is no question that stressful situations at school or within the family can play a role. If stressful factors are recognized to be present, counseling can be of value.

The pharmacologic management of migraine can be divided into (a) symptom control, (b) abortive measures, and (c) prophylactic treatment. Suppression of the patient's symptoms may include the use of analgesics orally, intramuscularly, or rectally, as well as the use of antiemetics and sedatives. In addition, modification of the environment by placing the patient in a dark, quiet room and applying cold compresses is reported to be useful. Narcotic analgesics generally are not needed. My personal practice is to treat the patient with rectal salicylates and tremethobenzamide. If a patient comes to the emergency room in the throes of a severe or prolonged attack, Raskin (48) has suggested using dihydroergotamine. Experience with this regimen in younger children is limited.

In the young patient with infrequent attacks (one per month), prophylactic medication usually is not indicated and abortive medication cannot be used since the patients usually do not have an aura, cannot be relied upon to take the medication sequentially, and are not allowed to take medications to school. In these patients, simple analgesics and antiemetics are useful. If, however, a young patient has frequent attacks—say, three or four times per month—and has missed a significant amount of school, prophylactic medications may be indicated. In an adolescent patient with frequent or infrequent attacks, if an aura is present, abortive medication, such as the ergot compounds or isometheptene mucate, should be used. Both of these medications constrict peripheral vessels and abort the migraine attacks. They do not seem to constrict intracranial vessels, nor do they seem to affect cerebral blood flow. These medications work best when taken at the initiation of the aura, before the onset of the severe pounding headache. The ergotamine compounds, although they cause nausea in some patients, can be used nasally, sublingually, orally, or rectally. In the adolescent with an aura, the patient is instructed to take ergotamine as an adult would. Analgesics and antiemetics can be given along with the ergotamine. Although ergotamine habituation is a problem in adults, it is not a problem in adolescents. Isometheptene mucate is given to adolescent patients in a fashion similar to its administration in adults. Antiemetics can be used at the same time. Instruction and reinstruction is necessary when using these medications in adolescent patients. These medications are not as effective when used in the adolescent without an aura. If either young patients or adolescent patients have frequent attacks, with or without an aura, or if abortive medications have been unsuccessful in the adolescent patient, prophylactic medications are quite useful. We attempt to use these medications over a four- to six-month period, completely relieving the patient's attack; then, we attempt to discontinue the medication. In many patients, once the attacks have been controlled for several months, they do not seem to recur when medication is discontinued. The medications employed most frequently in our pediatric neurology division include cyproheptadine, propranolol, and amitriptyline (49-51).

Cyproheptadine has both antihistamine and calcium-channel-blocking properties. It also is a serotonin antagonist. It is useful in patients who cannot take beta blockers. The usual dosage in an 8- to 16-year-old individual is 8 to 12 mg per day. I usually begin with 4 mg at bedtime and increase the dosage to 8 mg at bedtime after one week. I leave it at that dosage for several weeks and, if there is no improvement, usually prescribe 4 mg in the morning and 8 mg at bedtime. After six weeks, if there has been no improvement at all, the medication is not going to be effective. The major side effects of this medication are sedation and an

Migraine in Childhood

increased appetite. When cyproheptadine is used, the patient's weight must be monitored closely, since excessive weight gain is not uncommon.

Propranolol is known to be useful in adult migraine and is being used with increasing frequency in the treatment of migraine in children and adolescents. Having gained experience with this medication in pediatric cardiology, I use dosages in the range of 2 to 4 mg/kg. If the standard preparation is used, the medication should be given in a BID dosage. If the long-acting form is used, the medication can be taken once at night. Again, we start with a low dosage in the range of 10 to 20 mg h.s. and build it up by 10 to 20 mg every week or two until a dosage of 2 mg/kg is achieved. At this dosage, we monitor for side effects and watch the patient for four to six weeks. If the patient's attacks are successfully controlled at this dosage, we continue the medication for four to six months. If, however, the attacks are not controlled, the medication is increased gradually until the patient is taking 3 to 4 mg/kg. The patient should be watched for bradycardia, hypotension, sleep disorders (including nightmares), and depression; the latter can be quite severe. If the patient's attacks are controlled for four to six months, the dosage of medication is slowly tapered. If the attacks increase and become more severe, therapy may be resumed. Propranolol prevents arterial dilatation by blocking beta receptors. It also blocks catecholamine-induced platelet aggregation, decreases platelet adhesiveness, and prevents epinephrine release. It is contraindicated in patients with asthma or certain cardiac-conduction defects. An additional side effect may be decreased athletic tolerance.

Amitriptyline has been used in the treatment of migraine with or without associated depression, as well as in the mixed-headache syndrome. Treatment is initiated with 25 mg h.s. in the adolescent patient and slowly increased 50 to 200 mg as tolerated. Measurement of blood levels can be helpful and used as a guide to treatment, compliance, and the avoidance of toxicity. Side effects include dizziness, dry mouth, visual blurring, and urinary retention, but are rarer in children and adolescents than in adults. If significant depression accompanies the patient's headache, concomitant psychiatric treatment is indicated.

Calcium-channel-blocking agents currently are being tested in the treatment of migraine in adults. They should not be used routinely in the treatment of children unless primary modalities of treatment with which there is greater experience have been ineffective. These agents seem to work through their effect on smooth muscle and by prevention of vasoconstriction.

Nonsteroidal anti-inflammatory agents have been effective in some migraine patients, but have not been prospectively tested in children. They may have a special place in the treatment of menstrual migraine and exertional headache (52).

Anticonvulsants such as phenytoin and phenobarbital have been used for years to treat migraine. Well-documented studies include a double-blind protocol, and blood levels are not available. The adverse effects of these drugs on behavior in cognition make them inappropriate for primary use in the treatment of migraine headaches in children. In particularly resistant cases, methysergide can be considered; however, its well-known complications of pleural, cardiac, and retroperitoneal fibrosis prevent its chronic use. If the medication is used, a drug holiday should interrupt treatment every four to six months. The vast majority of children with migraine are responsive to treatment, and refractoriness often is due to incorrect diagnosis and is seen most frequently in patients with mixed-headache syndromes or daily muscle-contraction headaches (13).

PROGNOSIS

Data concerning the outcome of childhood migraine are inconclusive. Results of a longitudinal study conducted by Bille (53) in 73 children with pronounced migraine showed that 20% were free from migraine for at least two years during puberty or as young adults. Of these 73 patients, 22% had had migraine regularly since that time. By age 30, 40% were migraine-free—52% of the men and 30% of the women. At age 37 to 43, 53% of the patients continued to have migraine, with as many as 30% having had it continuously from childhood. Of men who reproduced, one-fourth had children with recurrent headaches. Of women with migraine, one-half had children with recurrent headaches. Hockaday (7) questioned whether it is ever safe to say that migraine has remitted completely, since 10 of her patients with migraine had been symptom-free for 4 to 10 years and then the headaches recurred. I agree that prolonged follow-up is ncessary before the outcome can be predicted, although I would say that about 15% may go into remission yearly and that boys ultimately have a better prognosis than girls. Matthew (32) describes an evolution from paroxysmal migraine in children and adolescents to mixed vascular-headache syndromes occurring daily in adults. It is not known whether prophylactic treatment of paroxysmal headache disorders in children and adolescents can prevent this evolution.

REFERENCES

1. Leviton, A. (1978). Epidemiology of headaches, *Advances in Neurology*, vol. 19 (B. S. Schoenberg, ed.), Raven Press, New York, pp. 341-353.
2. Friedman, A. P. The headache and history, literature, and legend, *Bull. NY Acad. Med., 48*: 661-681.
3. Day, W. H. (1873). *Essays on Diseases of Children*, Churchill, London.
4. Bille, B. S. (1962). Migraine in school children, *Acta Paediatr. Scand. (Suppl. 136), 51*: 1-151.
5. Friedman, A. P. and Harms, E. (1967). *Headaches in Children,* Charles C Thomas, Springfield, Illinois.
6. Barlow, C. F. (1984). Headaches and migraine in children, J. B. Lippincott, Philadelphia.
7. Hockaday, J. M. (1988). *Migraine in Childhood,* Butterworth, London.
8. Jay, G. W. and Tomasi, L. G. (1981). Pediatric headaches: A one-year retrospective analysis, *Headache, 21*: 5-9.
9. Goldstein, M. and Chen, T. C. (1982). The epidemiology of disabling headache, *Advances in Neurology*, vol. 33 (B. S. Schoenberg, ed.), Raven Press, New York, pp. 377-390.
10. Ad Hoc Committee on Classification of Headache (1962). Classification of headache, *JAMA, 179*: 717-718.

11. Proceedings of the Migraine and Headache Research Group, World Federation of Neurology, 1973.
12. Rothner, A. D. (1983). Diagnosis and management of headache in children and adolescents, Neurologic Clinics, Philadelphia. W. B. Saunders 1: 511-526, 1983.
13. Rothner, A. D. (xxxx). The migraine syndrome in children and adolescents, *Pediatric Neurology, 2*: 3.
14. Paine, R. S. and Oppe, T. E. (966). Neurological examination of children, *Clinics and Developmental Medicine, 20*: 21.
15. Kinast, M., Luders, H., Rothner, A. D., et al. (1982). Benign focal epileptiform discharges in childhood migraine, *Neurology, 32*: 1309-1311.
16. Liveing, E. (1873). *On Megrim, Sick Headache, and Some Allied Disorders: A Contribution to the Pathology of Nerve Storms*, Churchill, London.
17. Graham, J. R. and Wolff, H. G. (1938). Mechanisms of migraine headache and action of ergotamine tartrate, *Arch. Neurology and Psychiatry, 39*: 737-763.
18. Sicuteri, F. (1967). Vaso-neuroactive substances and their implication in vascular pain, *Research Clinic in the Study of Headache, 1*: 6-10.
19. Lauritzen, M., Olsen, T. S., Lassen, N. A., et al. (1983). Changes in regional blood flow during the course of classic migraine attacks, *Ann. Neurol., 13*: 633-641.
20. Kandt, R. S. and Levine, R. M. (1987). Headache and acute illness in children, *J. Child Neurology, 2*: 22-27.
21. Honig, P. J. and Charney, E. G. (1982). Children with brain tumor headaches, *Am. J. Dis. of Childhood, 136*: 99-100.
22. Friedman, A. P. et al. (1954). Migraine and tension headaches—a clinical study of two thousand cases, *Neurology, 4*: 773-778.
23. Prensky, A. L. and Sommer, D. (1979). Diagnosis and treatment of migraine in children, *Neurology, 29*: 506-510.
24. Carter, C. M., Egger, J., and Soothill, J. F. (1985). A dietary management of severe childhood migraine, *Human Nutrition—Applied Nutrition, 39A*: 294-303.
25. Menkes, M. M. (1974). Personality characteristics and family roles of children with migraine, *Pediatrics, 53*: 560-564.
26. Andrasik, F., Kabela, E., Quinn, S., et al. (1988). Psychological functioning of children who have recurrent migraine, *Pain, 34*: 43-52.

27. Dalsgaard-Nielsen, T. (1965). Migraine and hereditary, *Acta Neurologica Scand., 41*: 287-300.
28. Barabas, G., Matthews, W. S., and Ferrari, M. (1983). Childhood migraine and motion sickness, *Pediatrics, 72*: 188-190.
29. Barabas, G., Ferrari, M., and Matthews, W. S. (1983). Childhood migraine and somnambulism, *Neurology, 33*: 948-949.
30. Litman, G. I. and Friedman, H. M. (1978). Migraine and the mitral valve prolapse syndrome, *American Heart Journal, 96*: 610-640.
31. Rothner, A. D. (1988). "Comparing Childhood and Adult Migraine," Syllabus, American Academy of Neurologists 40th Annual Meeting, Cincinatti, Ohio, April 1988.
32. Matthew, N. T., Subitz, E., and Nigam, M. (1981). Transformation of migraine into daily headaches—analysis of factors, *Headache, 21*: 125-129.
33. Serdaru, M., Chrias, J., and Lhermitte, F. (1984). Isolated benign cerebrovasculitis or migrainous vasospasm, *J. Neurol. Neurosurg. Psychiatry, 47*: 73-76.
34. Bradshaw, P. and Parsons, M. (1965). Hemiplegic migraine and clinical study, *Quart. J. Med., 34*: 65-71.
35. Bickerstaff, E. R. (1964). Ophthalmoplegic migraine, *Review Neurologic, A110*: 582-584.
36. Bickerstaff, E. R. (1961). Basilar artery and migraine epilepsy syndrome, *Proc. Royal Society of Medicine, 55*: 167-169.
37. Dugan, M. C., Locke, S., and Gallagher, J. R. (1962). Occipital neuralgia in adolescents and young adults, *NEJM, 267*: 1166-1172.
38. Gascone, G. and Barlow, C. F. (1970). Juvenile migraine presenting as acute confusional state, *Pediatrics, 45*: 628-631.
39. Rothner, A. D., Erenberg, G., Cruse, R. P., et al. (1982). Acute aphasic migraine, *Headache, 22*: 150-151.
40. Prensky, A. L. (1976). Migraine and migrainous variants in pediatric patients, *Pediatric Clinics in North America, 23(3)*: 461-471.
41. Basser, L. S. (1964). Benign paroxysmal vertigo in childhood, *Brain, 87*: 141-142.
42. Deonna, T. and Martin D. (1981). Benign paroxysmal torticollis in infancy, *Arch. Diseases of Childhood, 56*: 956-957.
43. Casaer, L. I., Debeukalaar, F., and Amery, W. L. (1987). Flunarizine—a calcium entry blocker in childhood migraine, epilepsy and alternating hemiplegia, *Clinical Neuropharmacology, 10*: 162-168.

44. Kunkel, R. S. (1986). Acephalgic migraine, *Headache, 26*: 4, 198-201.
45. Haas, D. C. and Sovner, R. D. (1969). Migraine attacks triggered by mild head trauma and their relation to certain posttraumatic disorders of childhood, *J. Neruol. Neurosurg. Psychiatry, 32*: 548-554.
46. Anderman, N. F. and Lugaresi, E. (1987). *Migraine and Epilepsy*, Butterworth, Boston, pp.
47. Olness, K. N. and McDonald, J. T. (1987). Return headaches in children—diagnosis and treatment, *Pediatrics in Review, 8*: 307-311.
48. Raskin, N. H. (1986). Repetitive intravenous dihydroergotamine as therapy for intractable migraine, *Neurology, 36*: 995-997.
49. Bille, B., Ludbigsson, J., and Sannerg, G. (1977). Prophylaxis of migraine in children, *Headache, 17*: 61-63.
50. Ludvigsson, J. (1974). Propranolol used in prophylaxis of migraine in children, *Acta Neurologica Scand. 50*: 109-115.
51. Couch, J. R., Ziegler, D. K., and Hassaneim, R. (1976). Amitriptyline in the prophylaxis of migraine, *Neurology, 26*: 121-124.
52. Diamond, S. and Dalessio, D. J. (1986). *Practicing Physician's Approach to Headache*, 4th Ed., William & Wilkins, pp. 48-63.
53. Bille, B. (1982). Migraine in childhood, *Panminerva Medica, 24*: 57-62.

10

Biofeedback Therapy for Migraine

Frank Andrasik *University of West Florida, Pensacola, Florida*

Oliver N. Oyama* *The Avalon Center, Inc., Milton, Florida*

Russell C. Packard *Neurology and Headache Management Center and University of West Florida, Pensacola, Florida*

INTRODUCTION

Biofeedback as a treatment for migraine arose from an interesting mixture of basic research findings, clinical acumen, and serendipity. The biofeedback movement in general can be traced back to the 1960s, when a number of scientific findings and sociocultural trends began to converge (1). At this time, empirical studies (2–12) were beginning to show that both human and animal subjects could be conditioned to control certain autonomic nervous system functions, among these being blood pressure, salivation, gastrointestinal contractions, urine formation, sweat-gland activity,

---

Present affiliation: Duke/FAHEC Family Medicine Residency Program, Fayetteville, North Carolina

vasomotor response, and cardiac activity. The possibility that glandular and visceral responses, heretofore thought to function automatically and even unconsciously, could begin to be influenced by the conscious attempts of individuals opened the eyes of many medical visionaries. This possibility also fit well with a growing interest in exploring the boundaries of consciousness and altered states of awareness and in dealing more effectively with the adverse mental and physical effects of stress.

It was against this background that pioneering work was undertaken at the Menninger Clinic in Topeka, Kansas, to study psychophysiological variables in migraine patients. During a standard laboratory evaluation at this clinic, it was discovered in one patient that spontaneous termination of headache was accompanied by flushing in the hands and a rapid, sizable rise in surface hand temperature. This astute observation, combined with clinical creativity, led researchers there to pilot-test whether teaching migraineurs how to increase their peripheral temperature voluntarily might afford patients some improved ability to regulate their headaches. (It also led the researchers to contemplate at great length the theoretical mechanisms that might underlie this approach.) In early research conducted at Menninger (13–15), highly sensitive temperature probes were attached to a patient's index finger and to the middle of the forehead. The temperature differential between these two probes was displayed to the subjects, who then were instructed in ways to increase hand temperate relative to forehead temperature. This thermal biofeedback was combined with components of autogenic therapy, resulting in what was termed *autogenic feedback*.

Autogenic training has an extensive history (16) and involves having patients passively concentrate on key words and phrases selected for their ability to promote desired somatic responses. To facilitate increased blood flow to the extremities, which accounts for the peripheral warming effect, patients were instructed to focus on feelings of warmth and heaviness in the extremities (two of six components of autogenic therapy). Extensive practice in the laboratory and at home was necessary for patients to gain sufficient control of peripheral temperature to use the technique as a way to control headache. Initially, it was not known whether the temperature change occurring in patients was due to forehead-cooling, hand-warming, or both. Subsequent study revealed that most of the effect essentially was due to hand-warming, so most present-day biofeedback therapists monitor temperature from the hand alone. It is speculated that hand-warming derives its effect indirectly from the decreased SNS arousal that must occur for peripheral dilatation to occur, a notion that has gained support in the experimental literature (17,18).

In a subsequent follow-up assessment conducted on 74 patients who participated in an extensive course of the above-outlined treatment (spanning 270 days), Sargent et al. (19) found that 33 patients (45%) were improved by 51% or more; 22 patients (30%) obtained moderate improvement (26% to 50%); and 19 patients (25%) obtained slight or no improvement. Attrition was an acknowledged problem in this early, demanding investigation; 110 patients entered into the 270-day treatment and evaluation project, of whom 36 dropped out. Controls for expectancy, placebo, and similar effects were not incorporated into the design of this pilot work, but it is likely that such effects were minimal due to the heightened severity, chronicity, and prior resilience of most treated subjects.

Hand-warming biofeedback remains the predominant nonpharmacologic treatment for migraine, but a second type of biofeedback is being studied increasingly for vascular headache. This treatment procedure evolved from a more straightforward rationale and involves monitoring blood-volume pulse (BVP) from the temporal artery to teach patients how to reduce or constrict blood flow to the temporal region. The procedure may be thought of as the nondrug equivalent to ergotamine therapy. The initial effectiveness of this biofeedback treatment was evaluated by Friar and Beatty (20). Nineteen migraineurs, 18 of whom had reported prior treatment success with ergotamine tartrate, were carefully selected from a pool of 74 potential patients. Measures of blood flow were taken from pressure-transducing plethysmographs attached at two different sites—one directly above the temporal artery or to one of its main ramifications and the other to the ventral surface of the index finger. Subjects were matched carefully and assigned randomly to receive pulse-amplitude feedback from the temporal area (experimental group) or the finger (control group), both in the direction of decreased blood flow. At the completion of eight training sessions, experimental subjects were able to decrease blood flow in the temporal region by 20% during nonheadache periods. No significant changes in temporal blood flow occurred for the control subjects. Experimental subjects improved by approximately 45%, versus 14% improvement by control subjects.

BVP biofeedback is complex to implement. To illustrate, Friar and Beatty's procedure required repeated calculations of pulse amplitude, skin temperature, pulse rate, and pulse-propagation time, and simultaneous monitoring of and subsequent correction for muscle-activity artifact (through visual analysis and construction of a pulse-wave template from the previous session). Few clinicians have been able to duplicate such an elaborate biofeedback procedure. Recent advances in microcomputers and psychophysiological software-interpretive programs no doubt will lead to increased application of this useful biofeedback treatment procedure by clinicians.

It is not uncommon for hand-warming and BVP biofeedback to be combined with other approaches designed to aid patients in controlling or relaxing their aberrant physiology. The most frequently used procedure is relaxation therapy. A common relaxation technique has the patient engage in a systematic series of muscle-tensing and muscle-releasing exercises to achieve an increased awareness of muscle tightness and tension that then can lead to cultivation of an overall relaxed state. Relaxation training is similar to biofeedback, in that both are largely somatic interventions. One major difference is the focus of therapy. Biofeedback targets specific response systems, while relaxation targets the entire body ("rifle" versus "shotgun" approach). Relaxation approaches studied to date include both active techniques (Jacobson's progressive muscle-relaxation training) and passive techniques. (meditation, yoga, and autogenic exercises) (16,21,22). Direct feedback of muscle tension from electromyographic (EMG) monitors often is used to enhance relaxation therapy.

Biofeedback Therapy for Migraine

There are many studies evaluating the clinical efficacy of hand-warming, BVP, and relaxation therapies, either alone or in combination, which precludes their separate review. Since 1980, several different evaluations have been conducted of extant literature by a technique that allows diverse studies to be evaluated statistically in an integrated analysis, so that effect size and mean improvement levels averaged across studies can be determined. In this procedure, known as *meta-analysis*, an outcome for an entire group of patients receiving a common treatment in a research study becomes the unit of analysis. Hence, it is an analysis of results from studies rather than from individual patients.

Mean improvement levels from these meta-analyses are presented in Table 1. From this table, it is learned that (a) symptom improvement from autogenic feedback ranges from approximately 50% to 65%; (b) BVP biofeedback seems somewhat less effective overall; (c) in more recent studies, thermal biofeedback by itself has not been found to be as effective as was once thought (a decrease of approximately one-half); (d) relaxation therapy is similar in effectiveness to autogenic feedback; and (e) these nonpharmacological treatments all exceed the effects obtained from medical, psychological, and waiting-list control procedures. The finding of similar levels of improvement for biofeedback and relaxation training has led some researchers to conclude that these procedures may be interchangeable clinically and may operate through similar mechanisms. More recent research, employing aspects of treatment crossover designs, suggests that this is unlikely and that biofeedback may afford certain patients distinct advantages over relaxation therapy (26). This has led present-day researchers to begin to search for patient characteristics that will aid clinicians in matching patients to particular nonpharmacological treatments. More is said about this in a later section of the chapter.

Most of the studies included in the above-cited meta-analyses have limited their posttreatment evaluation period to brief intervals, typically to six months or less. Few studies have examined biofeedback treatment effectiveness for periods of one year and

TABLE 1 Mean Improvement Rates from Three Separate Meta-Analyses of Biofeedback and Relaxation Therapies for Migraine

Study	ATFB	THFB	REL	BVPFB	THFB+REL	MDCT	PTCT	WTLT
Blanchard et al. (17)	65.1	51.8	52.7	—	—	16.5	—	—
Holroyd (18)	—	28.1	44.4	—	57.4	—	—	11.0
Blanchard and Andrasik (19)	48.5	27.2	48.3	43.2	—	—	25.8	13.3

ATFB = Autogenic feedback or thermal biofeedback augmented by components of autogenic training, as developed at the Menninger Clinic
THFB = Thermal biofeedback by itself
REL = Relaxation therapy
BVPFB = Blood-volume-pulse biofeedback
MDCT = Medical control procedure; results taken from double-blind, placebo-controlled medication trials
PTCT = Psychological or pseudotherapy control procedure
WTLT = Waiting-list control procedure

beyond. Those that have, however, suggest that the initial effects do tend to endure (27-29).

BIOFEEDBACK IN RELATION TO MEDICAL THERAPY

Most patients who are seen for biofeedback treatment of headaches also are taking some form of prescription and/or over-the-counter medication. Many of these individuals are interested in biofeedback and related treatments because migraine medication is no longer effective, has adverse side effects, or costs too much. Sometimes, the continued use of analgesics and/or minor tranquilizers is associated with the problem of diminished treatment response and the development of tolerance and drug dependency. Many physicians and patients are considering biofeedback as an alternative treatment, either in conjunction with drug therapy or as an alternative that may be effective and safer (30).

If a patient believes that medication is still useful in relieving pain or preventing headache, it may be continued until the patient has achieved some degree of proficiency with biofeedback, before beginning a gradual withdrawal from the medications (31). Pharmacotherapy can be a useful adjunctive treatment with biofeedback and may be appropriate to continue, especially prophylactic medications (32). For instance, diazepam plus EMG feedback has been found to be more useful for reducing the anxiety of psychiatric patients than either one used alone (33). At other times, biofeedback may stand in for drugs in situations where sedatives may be either risky or contraindicated, yet the patient needs to be calmed. In some instances, a drug may need to be discontinued or tapered if it is interfering with the biofeedback learning (i.e., the patient is too tranquilized to focus on feedback).

Most of the subjects in biofeedback research studies do not appear to have been weaned from or stabilized on their existing medication routines. Thus, nearly all investigations of biofeedback actually may represent studies of biofeedback combined with uncontrolled use of medications (26). Only recently has research attempted to separate the interactive effects of medication in biofeedback treatment.

Two direct comparisons of biofeedback and medication for migraine have been reported, with different outcomes. Propranolol plus occasional analgesics were found to be similar in effectiveness to biofeedback combined with relaxation (34). Significantly more attrition occurred for the drug-therapy group, however. The same year, Mathew (35) compared biofeedback to abortive plus analgesic therapy, propranolol alone, amitriptyline alone, and various combinations of drugs and biofeedback for patients with migraine and mixed migraine-muscle-contraction headache. Five hundred and fifty-four patients out of an initial 800 completed all phases of the study. Biofeedback was found to be more effective than abortive-analgesic treatment for both headache types (see Table 2). The three regimens of prophylactic medication (propranolol alone, amitriptyline alone, and the two combined) exceeded biofeedback in most comparisons. Administering biofeedback concurrently with prophylactic medication appeared to enhance effectiveness by an additional 10% to 20%, supporting the utility of combining medical and biofeedback treatments. For both headache types, the greatest improvement occurred with the combination of some type of prophylactic medication and biofeedback.

Research suggests that there may be a problem with certain combinations of biofeedback and medication. For example, propranolol was found to impede the progress of migraine patients undergoing concurrent thermal biofeedback (36). Patients were able to reach established biofeedback training criteria, but with significantly greater difficulty and increased frustration. Beta-blocker-type medications are used widely for treatment of migraine, but no one has investigated whether other types of beta-blockers also might disrupt biofeedback training progress. In that the major mechanism of these drugs seem similar, one might suspect finding the same difficulty among patients. Jay et al. (36) noted similar interference for the tension-headache patients receiving EMG biofeedback while simultaneously taking amitriptyline. These findings are important to consider, because many other tricyclic-antidepressant medications have been found effective for

TABLE 2 Headache Improvement as a Function of Biofeedback and Medical Treatment—Data from Mathew (35)

Migraine Patients

Treatment condition	Number of patients completing treatment	Percentage of improvement
Medication control (ergotamine + analgesic)	33	20
Biofeedback	31	35
Amitriptyline	32	42
Amitriptyline + biofeedback	38	48
Propranolol	38	62
Propranolol + amitriptyline	38	64
Propranolol + amitriptyline + biofeedback	30	73
Propranolol + biofeedback	33	74

Mixed patients

Treatment condition	Number of patients completing treatment	Percentage of improvement
Medication control (ergotamine + analgesic)	35	18
Biofeedback	31	48
Propranolol	38	52
Amitriptyline	31	60
Propranolol + biofeedback	34	62
Amitriptyline + biofeedback	39	66
Propranolol + amitriptyline	36	69
Propranolol + amitriptyline + biofeedback	37	76

migraine prophylaxis. Although the mechanism of the antimigraine effect of propranolol has not been established, when beta-receptor sites are blocked, vasodilator responses to beta-adrenergic stimulation are decreased proportionately. This might make hand-warming (vasodilating) techniques more difficult to accomplish or take longer to learn in the presence of this medication. The mechanism of action for amitriptyline in prevention of migraine and of biofeedback learning is not known. Informing biofeedback patients about the potential interference of these types of medications might help to minimize frustration and offset lapses in patient motivation. Although we have not researched this systematically in our own work, we have encountered few difficulties in using biofeedback with patients taking the above medications, even in combination.

Biofeedback can be a useful adjunctive treatment in cases of medication abuse or overuse. One approach may be to have the patient eliminate analgesics gradually, while providing a concurrent course of relaxation or biofeedback (37,38). In the case of medication-rebound headache due to analgesics (39,40) and ergotamine preparations (40–42), it often is necessary to withdraw patients from these medications concurrently for effective treatment to be realized.

MECHANISMS OF BIOFEEDBACK THERAPY

While biofeedback is a relatively new therapeutic approach, it does have a strong theoretical basis, primarily in the area of learning. Consider the following traditional learning experiment. An animal is placed on a reinforcement schedule to shape a desired behavior. As the animal displays behaviors that approximate the desired behavior, it is reinforced with food pellets. The frequency of the reinforcement steadily increases as the animal displays behaviors that more closely approximate the desired behavior. Eventually, the animal learns to emit the desired behavior to obtain the reinforcer. You may recognize this behavioral-shaping experiment as an instrumental or "operant"-conditioning paradigm. This view emphasizes the antecedents and consequences (reinforcers) of behavior for its development and maintenance. In the context of biofeedback, the antecedents are the therapist's directions and encouragements for the patient to acquire a state of relaxation or autonomic control. Feedback of autonomic activity acts as the inherent reinforcer that then increases the frequency of the desired behavior. Learning theory is the basis for the oldest of the theoretical views of the mechanism of biofeedback and has received a considerable amount of support among psychophysiologists (as reviewed earlier).

Classical or Pavlovian conditioning, another of the learning theories, also has been suggested to explain the mechanism of biofeedback. Conditioning occurs when a physiological change is elicited by one stimulus and conditioned to occur in the presence of another, unrelated stimulus (the best known example being Pavlov's dogs, which were conditioned to salivate reflexively in response to a dinner bell). In this theoretical view, biofeedback is used as an assessment tool to determine when relaxation (the physiological change) occurs, so that a conditioned stimulus (e.g., cue relaxing word or relaxing mental image) can be applied. As Adler et al. (32) note, however, the mechanism of learning in this approach is primarily involuntary, and motivational variables are bypassed. Clearly, biofeedback involves motivational variables that lead to the acquisition of the desired behavior, lending this theory limited value.

The operant learning model, while quite strong in comparison to the classical conditioning model, also is limited, because it does not consider the role of cognitive or motivational contributions to behavior acquisition. Recent movement in the field of psychology and health sciences is toward a more integrated understanding of behavior to include not only overt variables, but also the interaction of overt variables with covert or cognitive variables. In the cognitive-behavioral model of biofeedback, beliefs, expectations, and the past learning history of patients are factored into behavioral change. Hence, the mechanism of biofeedback in this view incorporates not only the reinforcing elements of the feedback from both instrumentation and therapist, but also the desires, motivation, beliefs, and expectations that are addressed during traditional biofeedback therapy. As we will discuss in a later section, the instrumentation of biofeedback is only a part of the total treatment approach. Psychotherapeutic variables and conjoint treatment approaches are important elements of treatment outcome with biofeedback.

Finally, the last theoretical view involves what is termed a *skills-learning* orientation. In this approach, patients are seen as deficient in the skills, primarily relaxation or homeostasis of body and mind, necessary to cope with various psychophysiological problems. Biofeedback, then, assists the patient in developing, refining, or strengthening the skills needed to cope adaptively with internal and/or external stress. Biofeedback acts as an indicator of the patient's relative success in controlling the physical symptoms of stress.

CONSIDERATIONS IN SELECTING PATIENTS FOR TREATMENT

Many types of patients present for biofeedback: patients who have been frustrating to their physicians, those who have not been helped by traditional approaches, and those seeking a treatment that does not involve further medication. While certain patients who have been refractory to previous therapies can be helped with biofeedback, the tendency for patients with high motivation to have a better prognosis than their counterparts holds as true in biofeedback as it does in psychotherapy (43). In simple terms, the outcome relates directly to the time and motivation devoted to learning the biofeedback skills. Other variables bearing on treatment effectiveness are discussed below.

Age

Biofeedback can be used for patients of any age. Children and adolescents often take to biofeedback with enthusiasm, and many experience it as a kind of game (44). Decreased need for medication also has been reported among children with headache who have been trained with biofeedback (45). Diamond and Franklin

(46) term autogenic feedback the "best prophylactic-type therapy available" and the "treatment of choice in children with migraine" because of its heightened effectiveness with young patients. Interested readers are referred to Andrasik et al. (47) for a current review of biofeedback therapy with pediatric migraineurs.

Older patients often require more time to master biofeedback, and increased age has been correlated with a decreased response to biofeedback (28,48). Sargent et al. (15) speculated this to be the case in their early research and assumed that this was due chiefly to the increased rigidity that often accompanies increased age. Age is not an absolute barrier to the use of biofeedback, however, since some elderly people may learn the self-regulation quite well, but they may take a bit longer. Patient motivation may be a determining factor even in this group. It is important to be mindful of other factors in the elderly that can influence diagnosis or treatment: a higher prevalence of organic disease; the presence of cervical spine degenerative changes; the use of multiple medication regimens; and psychological factors such as loss-induced depression, a restricted life-style, or fear of dying.

Finding Time

Outcome in biofeedback treatment often depends on the patient's ability to find time to carry out and practice the treatment. Curiously, patients who cannot find time for biofeedback often are the ones who would benefit most from a self-regulatory type of treatment. Other patients may be looking for a quick fix in the shape of a pill or a new fad that will get rid of the headache. Still other patients may be managing their time quite well and truly have difficulty in finding time for biofeedback practice. These patients often can be helped with the suggestion of shorter periods of relaxation and/or biofeedback practice; the therapist may need to review the patient's schedule hour by hour to find times to insert important practice. Frequently, we see patients who have no awareness of their pace or the lack of time they devote to themselves until they actually try to become involved in biofeedback. This awareness in itself often can be very helpful in the overall management of the patient.

Frequency and Number of Sessions

Sessions usually are scheduled in the beginning for once or twice a week. Seeing patients twice a week initially often is most beneficial because it encourages them to practice outside of therapy, which is essential for success in the long run. Treatment length varies significantly from patient to patient and may be modifiable by many factors, including illness variables, patient variables, and therapeutic goals. Treatments typically range from 8 to 20 sessions. Patients with pathogenic headaches, with posttraumatic headaches, or whose headaches have proven long-standing and refractory may require longer treatment.

Personality Factors

It is important to conduct a routine mental-status examination with headache patients to rule out preexisting psychopathology that may compromise behavioral or self-regulatory treatments. Patients also should be given an explanation of the goal of biofeedback and how it works, because unrealistic expectations or fears about the time and commitment involved need to be dealt with early.

Perhaps the most common difficulty patients have with biofeedback is trying too hard to drive the feedback in the desired direction. Frustration may develop unless performance anxiety is minimized and a more passive strategy is adopted.

Many other psychological and personality factors become apparent during the course of biofeedback. If a patient repeatedly fails to practice, this should be recognized as a sign of resistance that needs exploration. It may mean poor motivation or that some important therapeutic issue is being overlooked.

Some patients may not practice or may not improve because of an unconscious reluctance to give up their symptoms. A not uncommon situation would be a patient who develops a disabling posttraumatic headache after suffering a mild blow to the head on the job. The patient may seem desperate to get better, yet does not practice and/or shows no improvement. This patient may, on an unconscious level, be reluctant to improve or lose the symptoms because this would leave the patient in a legally disadvantageous position for settling a claim with the insurance company. The patient also may be receiving secondary gain from a caring spouse, several physicians, or an eager attorney. These areas of resistance must be identified and discussed if they are to be resolved. Unfortunately, a number of these patients will angrily deny any such concerns or feelings and leave treatment altogether.

Once treatment has started, personality variables continue to play a role. Patients with histrionic personality disorder may become restless during sessions and neglect practice between sessions. Sometimes, they appear bored; at other times, they become frightened of their bodies and their impulses. A formal biofeedback approach in a well-lighted room may be helpful. The obsessive-compulsive patient often is diligent about home practice and may become frustrated at not meeting certain perfectionistic expectations. Such a patient may experience the feedback signal as criticism rather than as information. These difficulties may be minimized by using a low sensitivity setting on the feedback instrument, so that success at the task becomes easier, or by the therapist giving supportive verbal feedback about the direction of the change. Patients with character disorders usually have less anxiety or motivation for change, so they generally are less amenable to treatment.

Less Responsive Headache Types

Attempts to treat patients diagnosed as having cluster or menstrual migraine by biofeedback and related self-regulation treatments generally have proven to be unsuccessful (49–51). Occasionally, biofeedback and/or psychological therapy still may be of value to some of these patients by helping them to cope better with the psychological sequelae that often accompany repeated attacks of headache, which we term *headache-related distress*. Biofeedback also may be helpful for treating women whose migraines continue throughout pregnancy, when pharmacologic therapy options are necessarily limited.

Side Effects

In general, self-regulatory techniques have few serious contraindications or side effects. Patients have nothing added to their bodies to which they can become allergic. In fact, there are so few serious dangers associated with these techniques that the incautious professional can be lulled into unconcern about the problems that may occur. Temporary distortions of body image may occur during relaxation, an experience to avoid in borderline individuals or those who have experienced dissociative episodes. Patients who are extremely depressed, hypochondrical, or suffering from conversion symptoms generally do not do as well as patients who are aware of some anxiety and admit to some difficulty in knowing how to relax (32). Perhaps the primary caution is that the biofeedback technique should not be overvalued and viewed as a comprehensive treatment, but as a tool. It also is important not to apply these techniques at the wrong time, before more acute medical or psychiatric problems have been given full attention. A complete history and physical and neurologic examinations with appropriate tests always should be conducted first.

Nonspecific Benefits of Biofeedback

Important nonspecific benefits of both biofeedback and relaxation training have been observed in clinical practice (32). For instance, when a patient has fears or misconceptions about psychologists or psychiatrists, the time required to learn relaxation allows the patient to get to know the therapist and to reappraise the situation. Since biofeedback is viewed as a medical procedure, it allows the patient to save face during this introductory period. For the same reason, many physicians feel more comfortable referring patients for biofeedback than for psychotherapy. Biofeedback can provide a gentle introduction to psychological treatment for many unsophisticated or simply apprehensive patients. Andrasik et al. (27) inquired directly about positive and negative side effects experienced by headache patients one year after treatment with biofeedback and relaxation. Numerous positive side effects were reported; no subject attributed any harmful side effects to treatment.

The patient with long-standing problems may feel both helpless and hopeless. Biofeedback may allow patients to realize that even though they are unable to change all the stressors in their lives, they at least can influence their own reactions and in that way gain some autonomy from the stressors. Patients will learn to become more self-observant and may become more aware of the signals coming from their bodies, such as the need for rest, crying, touching, etc. As a patient's physical activity becomes quieted during the session, the patient may for the first time become aware of underlying resentments or other feelings.

Cost

Cost may be a consideration for the physician contemplating biofeedback for a patient. Cost also may be a matter of practical concern for patients themselves. At times, this has led to attempts to shortcut the teaching of relaxation by using less effective self-instruction techniques. One reason these techniques may not work as well is that if the patient concludes that the professional does not take the learning (and teaching) of relaxation seriously, why should the patient?

Researchers have begun to study whether the effectiveness of biofeedback and related self-regulatory interventions is compromised when administered in group settings, as one way to make these types of treatments more affordable. In early research we conducted (52,54), biofeedback usually was administered to two patients at once, primarily for reasons of convenience. Outcomes obtained from these two studies appeared to be similar to those obtained when biofeedback was administered individually, but no direct comparisons were attempted. More recently, Cote et al. (54) administered thermal biofeedback either individually or in a small-group format (groups composed of four to five patients) and found equivalent rates of improvement for their migraine patients.

A recent study (55) actually showed a general reduction in headache patients' medical expenses with biofeedback and relaxation treatment.

CONSIDERATIONS IN SELECTING BIOFEEDBACK THERAPISTS

Training and Credentials

The growing popularity of biofeedback in treating a variety of physiological as well as psychological disorders has led, as would be expected, to a significant increase in the number of professionals providing this service to the public. With the onslaught of biofeedback service providers comes the question for the physician, "Which provider do I send my patient to?" There are a few general issues to be aware of in making this selection. Biofeedback clinicians can be found in a variety of settings: mental-health centers, universities, medical schools, hospitals, and private practice. These clinicians hold degrees in psychology, social work, medicine, physical therapy, or related disciplines. Their training in biofeedback may have been formal, such as at one of the few professional training programs in the country, or as informal as a self-directed literature review. As the issue of reimbursement for biofeedback services has become more important, professionals are moving toward more formal training and credentialing in the area. Insurance companies and other reimbursement agencies are beginning to require credentialing in biofeedback, in line with their expectations for other modes of treatment. Credentialing for biofeedback service delivery exists at present through the Biofeedback Certification Institute of America, although credentialing currently is not required to provide the service. Despite the availablity of such credentialing, the physician should be aware that credentialing is not sufficient to imply competence in practice (56), although one could aruge that extended training and knowledge in the field would only add to a practitioner's competence.

A few suggestions in selecting a biofeedback provider include questioning the provider regarding certification, extended training (does the provider attend workshops or professional training

Biofeedback Therapy for Migraine

programs in the area of biofeedback?); academic pursuits involving biofeedback (does the provider present workshops or teach courses on biofeedback?); and, certainly, the professional standing in his or her specific field (e.g., licensing). We would recommend further that the physician informally discuss the provider's knowledge and competence in a personal meeting with the provider, since most biofeedback providers are eager to discuss the technique with someone from the medical profession, or invite the provider to present at an area medical association meeting or at medical rounds at an area hospital. These recommendations certainly would help to further broaden the understanding of this effective therapeutic technique, while facilitating collaboration in health care.

Therapist Characteristics and Variables

Despite the powerful therapeutic nature of the biofeedback technique, one must not neglect the mediating role of the therapist and the therapeutic relationship. While some therapists rely solely on the technique, it is our belief that biofeedback instrumentation is only one component of a more comprehensive self-regulatory intervention package.

One of the controversies in this area is the issue of whether the biofeedback therapist should be present or absent from the patient chamber. While our clinical intuition tells us that the presence of the therapist is desirable to provide therapeutic warmth, friendliness, and support (57), data indicate that excessive coaching by the therapist can be disruptive to patients (58). The experienced therapist knows when to leave the patient alone to practice biofeedback and when support and assistance would be valuable.

Another therapist variable that seems to affect treatment efficacy is the therapy rationale given to patients and the expectancy of success on the part of the patient. Greater clinical improvements have been found to occur when the therapist uses a convincing rationale and encourages the patient to understand the treatment procedures and participate actively in the treatment (59).

Finally, preparation of the patient for biofeedback by the referring physician, to include building the professional credibility of the biofeedback therapist, goes far to enhance therapeutic change. We cannot ignore the effects of placebo in the delivery of health-care services, and biofeedback is no exception. Patients who come to biofeedback believing in the technique and in the therapist who provides the service respond more favorably to biofeedback than do patients who are not prepared for therapy. Referring physicians need to reassure patients that the referral is *not* being made because the physician believes the problem is "psychological" or "all in your head," but rather as a way to address the physical problem (headache) in a more comprehensive fashion. Physicians may choose to provide an even more in-depth explanation of the treatment rationale. Packard (60) highlights the need that patients have for down-to-earth explanations for their discomfort, as well as for supportive and informative interactions with their physicians. This certainly can be applied to referrals for biofeedback therapy. Good "scripts" for the introduction of biofeedback to patients can be found in Andrasik (38), Blanchard and Andrasik (61), and Schwartz (56).

BIOFEEDBACK IN THE LARGER CONTEXT

Because of its strong somatic focus, biofeedback tends to be more readily accepted by patients than is traditional psychotherapy for stress management, since stress appears to play a role in the onset and exacerbation of headache in some migraineurs. Many patients find it difficult, if not impossible, to admit that a physical/somatic problem could derive from, or at least be maintained by, cognitive and behavioral variables. Because the instrumentation of biofeedback is physiologically based, it offers the patient an acceptable entré into behavioral therapy without having to deal with the strong stigma of such therapy. Furthermore, the novelty of biofeedback has brought many patients in for needed assessment and treatment who would not otherwise have come into the health-care system for their headaches.

Biofeedback Therapy for Migraine

Biofeedback rarely is conducted in isolation and, in fact, is more often part of a treatment package. Such a treatment package might include relaxation training, cognitive stress-coping skills training, family-marital counseling, and brief psychotherapy. Relaxation training can assist patients in dealing with stressful situations, and psychotherapy can lead to improvements in communication, problem solving, and general personal insights. Biofeedback patients frequently report improvements in other areas of their lives resulting from biofeedback therapy, and this may be due in part to this multicomponent approach. Case descriptions of the more typical combined treatment approach may be found in Andrasik (37) and Blanchard and Andrasik (61).

Sargent et al. (15) commented early on:

> An important trend is beginning to take place in the areas of psychosomatic disorders and medicine. This is the increasing involvement of the patient in his own treatment. The traditional doctor-patient relationship is giving way to a shared responsibility in which the patient is helped to become aware of this problems, both physical and emotional, and can therefore become a responsible partner in going toward psychosomatic and physical health. (page 427).

We look forward to the fulfillment of this promise in the care of migraine patients.

SUMMARY

Increasingly, biofeedback is being found useful in the treatment of migraine patients, either alone or in conjunction with medication. Considerations in selecting patients for biofeedback therapy should include headache diagnosis, motivation of the patient, personality, tolerance for medications, desire to avoid medications, frequency and severity of attacks, overall tension level, and willingness to practice between sessions. Sometimes, a brief trial of biofeedback can be useful for patients who at first may not see any connection between their worries and their physical symptoms or who show borderline motivation. Some of these patients may turn out to be well matched with biofeedback, or the assessment period may clarify the direction of treatment for the patient. It is important that clinicians administering biofeedback not only be familiar with current technologies, but also be experienced with other forms of therapy likely to be necessary to provide comprehensive care. Clinicians also should maintain close liaison with physician providers.

REFERENCES

1. Olson, R. P. and Schwartz, M. S. (1987). A historical perspective on the biofeedback field, *Biofeedback: A Practitioner's Guide* (M. S. Schwartz, ed.), Guilford Press, New York, pp. 3-16.
2. Engel, B. T. (1972). Operant conditioning of cardiac function: A status report, *Psychophysiology, 9*: 161-177.
3. Harris, A. H. and Brady, J. V. (1974). Animal learning—visceral and autonomic conditioning, *Annual Review of Psychology, 25*: 107-133.
4. Kamiya, J. (1969). Operant control of the EEG alpha rhythm and some of its reported effects on consciousness. In C.T. Hart (Ed.), *Altered states of consciousness: A book of readings*. New York: Wiley.
5. Kimmel, H. O. (1967). Instrumental conditioning of autonomically medited behavior. *Psychological Bulletin, 67*, 337-345.
6. Kimmel, H. O. (1979). Instrumental conditioning of autonomically mediated responses in human beings, *American Psychologist, 29*: 325-335.
7. Kristt, D. A., & Engel, B. T. (1975). Learned control of blood pressure in patients with high blood pressure. *Circulation, 51*, 370-378.
8. Miller, N. E. (1969). Learning of visceral and glandular responses, *Science, 163*: 434-445.
9. Miller, N. E. (1978). Biofeedback and visceral learning. *Annual Review of Psychology, 29*, 373-404.
10. Miller, N. E. and DiCara, L. (1967). Instrumental learning of heart rate changes in curarized rats: Shaping and specificity to discriminative stimulus, *J. Comparative & Physiological Psychology, 63*: 12-19.
11. Shapiro, D., Tursky, B., & Schwartz, G. E. (1970). Differentiation of heart rate and systolic blood pressure in man by operant conditioning. *Psychosomatic Medicine, 32*, 417-423.

12. Surwit, R. S., Shapiro, D., & Feld, J. L. (1976). Digital temperature autoregulation and associated cardiovascular changes. *Psychophysiology, 13,* 242-248.
13. Sargent, J. D., Green, E. E., and Walters, E. D. (1972). The use of autogenic feedback training in a pilot study of migraine and tension headaches, *Headache, 12:* 120-124.
14. Sargent, J. D., Green, E. E., and Walters, E. E. (1973). Preliminary report on the use of autogenic feedback training in the treatment of migraine and tension headaches, *Psychosomatic Medicine, 35:* 129-135.
15. Sargent, J. D., Walters, E. D., and Green, E. E. (1973). Psychosomatic self-regulation of migraine headaches, *Seminars in Psychiatry, 5:* 415-428.
16. Schultz, J. H. and Luthe, W. (1969). *Autogenic Training* (vol. 1), Grune & Stratton, New York.
17. Dalessio, D. J., Kunzel, M., Sternbach, R., and Sovak, M. (1979). Conditioned adaptation-relaxation in migraine therapy, *JAMA, 242:* 2102-2104.
18. Sovak, M., Kunzel, M., Sternbach, R., and Dalessio, D. J. (1978). Is volitional manipulation of hemodynamics a valid rationale for biofeedback therapy of migraine? *Headache, 18:* 197-202.
19. Sargent, J. D., Taylor, J. B., Coyne, L., Thetford, P. E., Walter, E. D., and Sergerson, J. A. (1975). Autogenic feedback in migraine headaches, *J. Kansas Med. Soc., 76:* 266-267.
20. Friar, L. R. and Beatty, J. (1976). Migraine: Management by trained control of vasoconstriction, *J. Consulting & Clinical Psychology, 41:* 46-53.
21. Benson, H., Klemchuk, H. P., and Graham, J. R. (1974). The usefulness of the relaxation response in the therapy of headache, *Headache, 14:* 49-52.
22. Warner, G. and Lance, G. W. (1975). Relaxation therapy in migraine and chronic tension headache, *Med. J. Australia, 1:* 298-301.
23. Blanchard, E. B., Andrasik, F., Ahles, T. A., Teders, S. J., and O'Keefe, D. (1980). Migraine and tension headache: A meta-analytic review, *Behavior Therapy, 11:* 613-631.
24. Holroyd, K. A. (1986). Recurrent headache, *Self-Management of Chronic Disease: Handbook of Clinical Interventions and Research* (K. A. Holroyd and T. L. Creer, eds.), Academic Press, Orlando, pp. 373-413.

25. Blanchard, E. B. and Andrasik, F. (1987). Biofeedback treatment of vascular headache, *Biofeedback: Studies in Clinical Efficacy* (J. P. Hatch, J. G. Fisher, and J. D. Rugh, eds.), Plenum, New York, pp. 1-79.
26. Andrasik, F. (1989). Biofeedback Applications for Headache, *Clinical Perspectives on Headache and Low Back Pain* (C. Bischoff, H. C. Troue, and H. Zenz, eds.), Hogrefe and Huber, Lewiston, NY, pp. 181-200.
27. Andrasik, F., Blanchard, E. B., Neff, D. F., and Rodichok, L. D. (1984). Biofeedback and relaxation training for chronic headache: A controlled comparison of booster treatments and regular contacts for long-term maintenance, *J. Consulting & Clinical Psychology, 52*: 609-615.
28. Diamond, S. and Montrose, D. (1984). The value of biofeedback in the treatment of chronic headache: A four-year retrospective study, *Headache, 24*: 59-69.
29. Knapp, T. W. (1982). Treating migraine by training in temporal artery vasoconstriction and/or cognitive behavioral coping: A one-year follow-up, *J. Psychosomatic Research, 26*: 551-557.
30. Billings, R. F., Thomas, M. R., Rapp, M. S., Reyes, E., and Leith, M. (1984). Differential efficacy of biofeedback in headache, *Headache, 24*: 211-215.
31. Budzynski, T. (1979). Biofeedback strategies in headache treatment, *Biofeedback—Principles and Practice for Clinicians* (J. V. Basmajian, ed.), Williams & Wilkins, Baltimore, pp. 132-152.
32. Adler, C. S., Adler, S. M., and Packard, R. C. (1987). The psychological use of biofeedback and other self-regulatory techniques in headache treatment, *Psychiatric Aspects of Headaches* (C. S. Adler, S. M. Adler, and R. C. Packard, eds.), Williams & Wilkins, Baltimore, pp. 349-368.
33. LaValle, Y. J., Lamontagne, Y., Pinard, G., et al. (1977). Effects of EMG feedback, diazepam, and their combination on chronic anxiety, *J. Psychosomatic Research, 21*: 65-71.
34. Sovak, M., Kunzel, M., Sternbach, R. A., and Dalessio, D. J. (1981). Mechanism of the biofeedback therapy of migraine: Volitional manipulation of the psychophysiological background, *Headache, 21*: 89-92.
35. Mathew, N. T. (1981). Prophylaxis of migraine and mixed headache. A randomized controlled study, *Headache, 21*: 105-109.
36. Jay, G. W., Renelli, D., and Mead, T. (1984). The effects of propranolol and amitriptyline on vascular and EMG biofeedback training, *Headache, 24*: 56-69.
37. Andrasik, F. (1985). Tension headache, *Behavior Therapy Casebook* (M. Herson and C. J. Last, eds.), Springer, New York, pp. 118-131.

38. Andrasik, F. (1986). Relaxation and biofeedback for chronic headaches, *Pain Management: A Handbook of Psychological Treatment Approaches* (A. D. Holzman and D. C. Turk, eds.), Pergamon, New York, pp. 213-239.
39. Kudrow, L. (1982). Paradoxical effects of frequent analgesic use, *Headache: Physiopathological and Clinical Concepts: Advances in Neurology* (vol. 33) (M. Critchley, A. Friedman, S. Gorinin, and F. Sicuteri, eds.), Raven Press, New York, pp. 335-341.
40. Worz, R. (1983). Analgesic withdrawal in chronic pain treatment, *Perspectives in Research on Headache* (K. A. Holroyd, B. Schlote, and H. Zenz, eds.), Hogrefe, Toronto, pp. 137-144.
41. Saper, J. R. (1987). Ergotamine dependency: A review, *Headache, 27*: 435-438.
42. Saper, J. R. and Jones, J. M. (1986). Ergotamine dependency, *Clinical Neuropharmacology, 9*: 244-256.
43. Adler, C. S. and Adler, S. M. (1979). Strategies in general psychiatry, *Biofeedback—Principles and Practice* (J. V. Basmajian, ed.), Williams & Wilkins, Baltimore, pp. 180-196.
44. Attanasio, V., Andrasik, F., Burke, E. J., Blake, D. D., Kabela, E., and McCarran, M. S. (1985). Clinical issues in utilizing biofeedback with children, *Clinical Biofeedback and Health, 8*: 134-141.
45. Werder, D. and Sargent J. (1984). A study of childhood headache using biofeedback as a treatment alternative, *Headache, 24*: 122-126.
46. Diamond, S. and Franklin, M. (1975). Biofeedback: Choice of treatment in childhood migraine, *Therapy in Psychosomatic Medicine* (vol. 4) (W. Luthe and F. Antonelli, eds.), Autogenic Therapy, Rome, pp. 190-192.
47. Andrasik, F., Blake, D. D., and McCarran, M. S. (1986). A biobehavioral analysis of pediatric headache, *Child Health Behavior: A Behavioral Pediatrics Perspective* (N. A. Krasnegor, J. D. Arasteh, and M. F. Cataldo, eds.), Wiley, New York, pp. 394-434.
48. Blanchard, E. B., Andrasik, F., Evans, D. D., and Hillhouse, J. (1985). Biofeedback and relaxation treatments for headache in the elderly: A caution and a challenge, *Biofeedback and Self-Regulation, 10*: 69-73.
49. Blanchard, E. B., Andrasik, F., Jurish, S. E., and Teders, S. J. (1982). The treatment of cluster headache with relaxation and thermal biofeedback, *Biofeedback and Self-Regulation, 7*: 185-191.
50. Solbach, P., Sargent, J., and Coyne, L. (1984). Menstrual migraine headache: Results of a controlled, experimental, outcome study of nondrug treatments, *Headache, 24*: 75-78.

51. Szekely, B., Botwin, D., Eidelman, B. H., Becker, M., Elman, N., and Schemm, R. (1986). Nonpharmacological treatment of menstrual headache: Relaxation-biofeedback behavior therapy and person-centered insight therapy, *Headache, 26*: 86-92.
52. Andrasik, F. and Holroyd, K. A. (1980). A test of specific and nonspecific effects in the biofeedback treatment of tension headache, *J. Consulting & Clinical Psychology, 48*: 575-586.
53. Holroyd, K. A., Andrasik, F., and Noble, J. (1980). A comparison of EMG biofeedback and a credible pseudotherapy in treating tension headache, *J. Behavioral Medicine, 3*: 29-39.
54. Cote, G., Gauthier, J., and Cote, A. (1986). "The Treatment of Migraine Headache: A Comparison of Group Versus Individual Biofeedback Training," paper presented at Twentieth Annual Meeting of the Association for the Advancement of Behavior Therapy, Chicago, Illinois.
55. Blanchard, E. B., Jaccard, J., Andrasik, F., Guarnieri, P., and Jurish, S. E. (1985). Reduction in headache patients' medical expenses associated with biofeedback and relaxation treatments, *Biofeedback and Self-Regulation, 10*: 63-68.
56. Schwartz, M. S. (1987). *Biofeedback: A Practitioner's Guide*, Guilford Press, New York.
57. Taub, E. and School, P. J. (1978). Some methodological considerations in thermal biofeedback training, *Behavioral Research Methods and Instrumentation, 10*: 617-622.
58. Borgeat, F., Hade, B., Larouche, L. N., and Bedwani, C. N. (1980). Effects of therapist active presence on EMG biofeedback training of headache patients, *Biofeedback and Self-Regulation, 5*: 275-282.
59. Shaw, E. R. and Blanchard, E. B. (1983). The effects of instructional set on the outcome of a stress management program, *Biofeedback and Self-Regulation, 8*: 555-565.
60. Packard, R. C. (1979). What does the headache patient want? *Headache, 19*: 370-374.
61. Blanchard, E. B. and Andrasik, F. (1985). *Management of Chronic Headaches: A Psychological Approach*, Pergamon Press, New York.

11

Migraine—Unproven Therapeutic Measures

Richard C. Peatfield* *St. James University Hospital, Leeds, England*

INTRODUCTION

It is inevitable that this chapter should be a catalog of disconnected observations, few of which (almost by definition) are supported by much scientifically acceptable evidence. While this review will try to be critical, much of the material is too diffuse even for this.

FEVERFEW

As its name implies, the leaves of the feverfew plant (Tanacetum or Chrysanthemum parthenium) (Figure 1), a native of the Balkan peninsula, have been used as a febrifuge since the Middle Ages and as a folk remedy for migraine for many years. Johnson (1) surveyed 300 migraine patients who admitted eating fresh leaves in sandwiches, crushed with honey or as icing sugar pills. The average

---
**Present affiliation*: Charing Cross Hospital, London, England

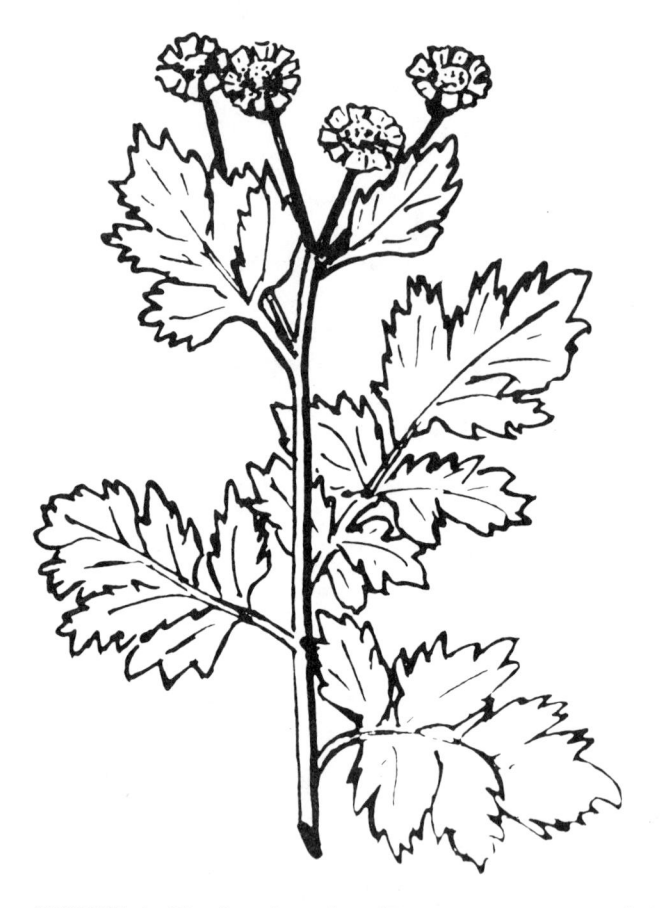

FIGURE 1 The feverfew plant (Tanacetum parthenium) (by courtesy of Dr. Stewart Johnson and the Sheldon Press).

dosage was two to four small or one to two large leaves daily, which is approximately equivalent to 60 mg of dried leaf, though commercially available dried leaf is of variable potency (2). Seventy percent of these subjects claimed that their attacks were less frequent or less severe, with 33% completely relieved; 30% were not helped. Four out of five patients who stopped taking the plant had a recurrence of severe migraine after two to three weeks (1,3). Johnson et al. (4,5) have published a double-blind trial of

17 such patients who had been taking feverfew with apparent benefit. Nine of these patients were given capsules containing inactive leaves on a double-blind basis, while 8 continued freeze-dried feverfew powder. The patients receiving placebo had a significant increase in frequency and severity of headache (Table 1) with nausea and vomiting, while those who continued to use feverfew were unchanged. Two patients taking placebo withdrew from the study to resume raw feverfew leaves. In another center, however, 30 patients were given feverfew without apparent benefit (6).

More recently, Murphy et al. (7) have reported a prospective double-blind trial of feverfew prophylaxis in 72 volunteers with migraine who were given dried leaf equivalent to two fresh leaves per day for four months, or matching cabbage placebo. Results were available for 59 of these volunteers. There was a significant (24%) reduction in the number of attacks during active feverfew treatment and a trend to less severe attacks, but no change in their duration. In two separate global assessment ratings, feverfew was superior to placebo ($p < .001$), and side effects were minimal.

There have been a number of reported side effects with feverfew treatment, including contact dermatitis (3) and cytotoxicity (8). In Johnson's earlier survey (1) 12% of subjects encountered soreness of the mouth, which sometimes necessitated stopping the treatment.

TABLE 1 Double-Blind Study of Feverfew in Migraine (4)

	n	Before taking feverfew	Upon taking feverfew	During study
Patients continuing feverfew	8	7.44	1.63	1.69
Patients given placebo	9	3.94	1.22*	3.13*

No. of attacks monthly

*These figures significantly differ, $p < .02$. Differences in headache frequency *between* the groups were significant for the last three months of the trial.

The active ingredient of feverfew has not yet been unequivocally identified—the leaves are rich in sesquiterpine lactones such as Parthenolide (Figure 2), which constitute about 0.87% of the dry weight and are believed to be responsible for the contact dermatitis. Extracts of feverfew appear to reduce the synthesis of prostaglandins by inhibiting phospholipase A (9-11). This contrasts with NSAIDs such as aspirin, which inhibit cyclo-oxygenase, the next enzyme in this pathway. Although feverfew extracts will reduce platelet degranulation and serotonin release in vitro (12, 13), platelet aggregation in vivo does not seem to be affected (14).

Heptinstall (13,15) attempted to isolate the components responsible for the platelet-inhibiting effect using chromatographic techniques. Five active sesquiterpine lactones were identified, of which Parthenolide was the most potent in this pharmacological model. The researchers thought that this action was mediated partly by inhibition of phospholipase A and partly by neutralizing sulphydryl groups on other enzymes involved in platelet aggregation and degranulation (16).

Clearly, expensive chronic-toxicity studies are required before either the leaf or any purified constituent can be introduced into clinical practice. The identification of any such compound requires an in vitro pharmacological system that may or may not turn out to be a valid model for migraine; yet, one cannot test a compound in migraine patients until its safety can be ensured.

We may, indeed, ultimately establish that the active constituent of feverfew has novel pharmacological properties that provide

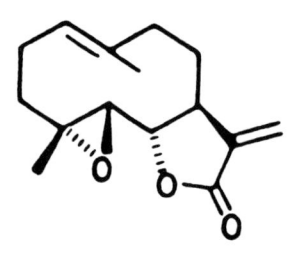

FIGURE 2 Chemical structure of Parthenolide

Unproven Therapeutic Measures

a clue to the pathophysiology of migraine itself. On the other hand, feverfew may turn out to share the limited efficacy and side effects of established nonsteroidal drugs such as aspirin.

AIR IONIZATION

Many patients associate their headaches with changes in the weather, especially with thunderstorms and the various hot dry winds that occur periodically in many countries (Table 2). These headaches are known to be accompanied by an increase in the number of small ionized particles in the air (Table 3) and with a greater proportion of ionized particles that are positively charged (18).

High concentrations of negatively charged ion particles, in contrast, are found near waterfalls and in coastal and alpine conditions (17). The association of positive ions with headache and general malaise and of negative ions with well-being led to the development in the 1950s of small electrical devices that deliver negative ions into a room. Unfortunately, most of the human studies with such devices have been performed poorly and often are inconclusive (19). Nevertheless, in one crossover study (18) of 129 subjects with headache, palpitations, dyspnoea, asthma, flushes, and vasomotor rhinitis, 96 reacted favorably to a negative ionizer, and only 16 of these reacted to positive ionization as well. Unfortunately, it is not clear from this report to what extent the objectives of the study were concealed from the subjects and how these symptoms were rated. Hawkins, in a double-blind study (20) of 38 subjects working in an insurance company office, also showed a reduction of headache prevalence from 16.5% to 5.5% when continuous negative ionization was employed. Human reaction times and EEG rhythms, however, are not affected by exposure to negative ions (19).

The biological effects of charged ions are not well understood—there is some evidence that positive ions increase and negative ions decrease platelet serotonin levels and the excretion of its metabolite 5HIAA in urine (21,22). However, one study (23) in rats demonstrated, paradoxically, that positive ions increased the

TABLE 2 "Winds of ill repute" Associated with Positive Ionization of the Atmosphere (17)

Chamsin or Sharav of the Middle East
Chinook of Canada
Desert winds of Arizona
Foehn of the European Alps
Mistral or Autun of France
North Winds of Melbourne, Australia
Santa Ana of California
Sirocco of Italy
Thar of India
Xlokk of Malta
Zonda or Xonda of Argentina

pain threshold. This effect was reversed by reducing serotonin levels with parachloro-phenylalanine, which suggests that it is mediated by enhancing central serotonin pathways.

BUILDING SICKNESS

Many workers attribute such symptoms as headache, lethargy, nasal stuffiness, chest tightness, and eye irritation to the atmosphere in the sealed air-conditioned offices they have to work in,

TABLE 3 Typical Concentrations of Ions/cc of Air

	+ve	−ve	Reference
Clear country air	1200	1000	25
Before Jerusalem Sharav	4500	4000	18
Naturally ventilated offices	185	177	24
Air-conditioned offices	342	256	
With negative-ion generators	–	1841	26

calling it "building sickness." In a systematic study, Robertson et al. (24) compared workers in two adjacent buildings, one ventilated naturally and one ventilated artificially. Seventeen out of 112 (15%) of the workers in the natural environment and 40 out of 129 (31%) in the air-conditioned environment complained of headache, and a significantly higher proportion of subjects in the air-conditioned offices complained of many of the other symptoms of building sickness. The temperature, humidity, concentrations of both negative and positive ions, and the ozone and formaldehyde levels were similar in the two environments, and no single mechanism for building sickness could be advanced (24,25). In a smaller study (26) of 26 subjects working in such a building, the authors failed to demonstrate any statistically significant benefit from negative-ion generators placed in each room, and other studies (25) also have been contradictory. Some of the symptoms may be due to the dispersal of pathogenic microorganisms by the ventilator system or to a genuine allergy to their antigens dispersed from the sludge that forms inside humidifiers (25,27).

It must be concluded that the association of symptoms such as headache with changes in the level of small air ions may be coincidental, and we await convincing systematic studies suggesting that artificially altering the ions in the atmosphere is in any way beneficial.

FOOD ALLERGY

About 18% to 19% of patients attending a specialized migraine clinic consider themselves sensitive to cheese and/or chocolate, and 11% are sensitive to citrus fruit (28,29). In this survey, 29% of patients reported sensitivity to alcoholic drinks, and about two-fifths of these were sensitive only to red wine, port, or sherry. The role of dietary precipitation in the pathogenesis of headache is discussed at length in several recent publications (29–33). There is no direct evidence that dietary precipitation is mediated by classical antigen-antibody reactions, and it seems more likely that some chemical constituent of these incriminated foods is responsible. Tyramine has been suggested, though experimental studies (30) in humans have not always been consistent. While there is no evidence that amine oxidation is deficient in dietary migraine patients (34), two independent research groups (35,36) have demonstrated a deficiency of one type of phenolsulfotransferase in platelets from the minority of diet-sensitive patients. This preferentially inactivates phenolic compounds other than tyramine, and it is thought that flavinoid compounds (for example, in red wine) may be the principal substrate for the enzyme (37). One always must bear in mind that 80% of migraine patients are able to consume these foods with impunity, so this biochemical mechanism cannot be in any way fundamental to the mechanism of the headache itself, but instead merely acts as one of a number of potential triggers for it.

Patients who have identified themselves as food-sensitive usually will have eliminated the incriminating substance from their diets long before seeking medical advice. There have been many clinical studies purporting to demonstrate that modifications to the diets of unselected migraine patients will ameliorate their headaches (for example—38,39). None of these studies are wholly convincing, largely because they were not properly blinded, and the subjects, often desperate for a cure, were particularly prone to placebo responses as a result of the undoubted enthusiasm of the physician in charge of the study. Only Egger's trial (40) has so far made any attempt to eliminate this effect, and this study was not performed on a wholly typical group of migrainous children (29, 33). All these trials are best seen as attempts to explore the pathogenesis of the headache, rather than demonstrations of a mode of treatment that can be of more general application.

HYPOGLYCEMIA

About 25% of children seeking advice about headaches associate attacks with a missed meal (41), and migraine is rare among diabetics (42), often settling as patients develop diabetes and recurring during episodes of hypoclycemia (43). Migraine attacks seem to follow insulin-induced hypoglycemia very rarely (44), however, which has led to the suggestion that attacks are related more to

Unproven Therapeutic Measures

stress than to hypoglycemia per se (45). While avoidance of hypoglycemia may benefit diabetic patients who continue to have headaches, these observations would appear to have few practical consequences for migraine subjects in general.

TREATMENT OF NECK STRUCTURES

Patients with a history of injuries to the neck or with pain in moving or touching the neck often complain of bilateral pain that even may be referred to the frontal region. It is believed that this distribution of referred pain is due not only to overlap in the cutaneous distribution of the trigeminal and cervical nerves (46), but also to the entry zones of the upper cervical roots, which supply the damaged parts of the cervical spine, being at the same levels of the cord as the descending tract of the trigeminal nerve (46–50). Many of these patients exhibit widespread degenerative changes on neck X-rays and respond to rest, with or without a collar, and NSAIDs.

Some patients complain of a much less diffuse, lateralized pain confined to the part of the occiput supplied by the third occipital nerve (C2-3). This pain has been attributed to osteoarthritic changes in the C2-3 zygo-apophyseal joints, which are supplied by twigs from these nerve roots (51). Relief can be obtained by blocking the root with local anesthetic, which may be followed by radio-frequency thermocoagulation. Some patients experience temporary light-headedness or ataxia due to loss of proprioceptive afferents from the neck.

Unilateral arthritis of the C1-2 lateral articulation, which is demonstrable on a CT scan, also can cause retromastoid pain in a more lateral distribution than that caused by the third occipital nerve. This pain can be relieved by local anesthetic injected into the joint or ganglion, which may be followed by C2 dorsal root section (52). One or both of the lateral atlanto-axial joints may be injured, for example, when the patient is in a car that is struck from behind. This type of injury may be associated with referred occipital pain radiating to the vertex, in the distribution of one or both of the greater occipital nerves. Bogduk (53,54) has obtained good results in such patients by using local anesthetic blockade of the C2 ganglia on one or both sides. In a controlled trial of 61 patients with whiplash injuries (55), early active mobilization was shown to be superior to rest in a cervical collar.

The convergence of nerves from the scalp and neck in the upper cervical cord has led to attempts to offer treatment directed at abnormalities in the neck to patients with typical migraine. Clearly, there is an overlap between migraine patients and those with the neck syndromes described above; nevertheless, most neurologists would exclude patients with unilateral occipital pain that is increased by neck movement from being classified as having common migraine. Bogduk (53) found that blockade of the C2 ganglion with local anesthetic was ineffective in common migraine. In contrast, Anthony (56) has obtained good results in patients with migraine and with cluster headache, as well as with occipital neuralgia, by injecting 160 mg of depot methylprednisolone into the region of the greater occipital nerve. Nineteen out of 20 patients with occipital neuralgia improved for a mean of 48 days, 18 out of 29 with cluster headache for a mean of 20 days, and 18 out of 20 with unilateral migraine for 30 days (range 13 to 66 days). Anthony (56) believes that the steroid induces local demyelination of this nerve. The mechanism of the pain relief is as yet unclear, but it may relate to a reduction in afferents contributing to the input to the cervical cord. Single neurons in related dorsal root ganglia may send divergent axons to the greater occipital nerve and to pain-sensitive blood vessels in the scalp or dura. Anthony does not feel that the steroid contributes by denervating the facet joints or the vertebral artery.

Parker et al. (57) reported a randomized, though not fully blind, trial of cervical manipulation in migraine. Eighty-five patients were divided into three groups. Twenty-three patients received twice weekly cervical manipulation, beyond the normal range of movements, by a doctor or physiotherapist. Thirty patients were given similar manipulation by a chiropractor, and 20 control patients were given small oscillatory movements ("mobilization") by a doctor or physiotherapist. All three groups improved after the two-month treatment phase, but there were no statistically significant differences in outcome among the three groups.

TEMPOROMANDIBULAR JOINT DISEASE

Removal of upper and lower molar teeth can result in overclosure of the jaw, putting strain on the temporomandibular joint that may be reflected in clicks and recognizable joint pain (58,59). Such patients often benefit from dental appliances that restore the normal range of jaw movements (59). Nevertheless, significant numbers of patients with facial pain have normal temporomandibular joint anatomy, and overclosure is common in pain-free control subjects (59). While this pain occasionally can radiate into the temples, there is very little evidence that headache can be so mediated, and even less that altering apparently normal jaw closure will confer benefit on patients complaining of any type of jaw, face, or head pain. A trial of dental occlusive therapy, for example, in consecutive patients complaining of "atypical facial pain" proved negative (60). These patients seemed to benefit more from antidepressant medication, whether they fulfilled research criteria for depression or not.

MANIPULATION OF PLASMA LIPIDS

Leviton and Camenga (61) reported classic migraine in two achondroplastic brothers with hyperprebetalipoprotaeinaemia; the attacks ceased almost completely in the more severely affected brother once the lipid levels were reduced by clofibrate. These authors speculated that the mechanism may relate to changes in blood viscosity or to platelet clumping.

More recently, Glueck and Bates (62) found levels of low-density lipoprotein (LDL) cholesterol above the 90th percentile in 9 out of 26 boys (aged 4 to 20) with severe migraine. This is a significantly greater proportion than predicted ($p < .01$). In 11 out of 39 families, there was a family history of premature myocardial infarction or stroke involving grandparents or parents, and in 3 out of 9 families, there was a first-degree relative with LDL cholesterol above the 90th percentile. There were correspondingly low levels of high-density lipoprotein (HDL) in 6 patients. This may relate either to platelet hyperaggregability or to alterations of endothelial prostaglandin metabolism.

A double-blind, crossover trial of fish oil, which is rich in omega-3 fatty acids, was performed in 15 refractory migraine patients and reported in abstract form by Glueck et al. (63). It must be recorded, however, that Glueck's research work has come under recent adverse scrutiny (64). In Glueck's study, headaches were significantly less intense when subjects took capsules containing 15 g of fish oil daily for six weeks, by comparison to placebo oleate-linoleate capsules. Clinical benefit seemed to parallel changes in red-cell membrane lipid composition and a decrease in platelet serotonin release, though the primary effect may be to direct prostaglandin pathways toward the less pro-inflammatory three series prostaglandins, most notably the thromboxanes (65).

ACUPUNCTURE

Despite its widespread use since its introduction in the West from China, there have been few systematic, controlled studies of acupuncture in headache patients. Loh et al. (66) reported a crossover trial of acupuncture in 48 refractory migraine and tension headache patients; unfortunately, only 29 of these received both forms of treatment, because 12 out of 25 given acupuncture first, and 7 out of 25 given medical treatment first, refused to change. A total of 41 patients received acupuncture, of which 24 improved. Thirty-six patients had a further course of various prophylactic drugs (most commonly propranolol), and 9 improved. Patients with local tender spots on the head and neck were more likely to benefit from the acupuncture. Clearly, the highly selected patients recruited into this trial, and the violations of the planned protocol, do not permit a valid comparison between any single prophylactic drug and acupuncture.

Dowson et al. (67) performed a single-blind comparison of a course of six weekly treatments with either mock transcutaneous nerve stimulation or genuine acupuncture in 48 patients with common or classic migraine drawn from a British general practice. Fourteen out of 25 patients (56%) in the acupuncture group and 7 out of 23 (30%) receiving mock stimulation obtained 33% greater pain relief in the four weeks after the end of the active treatment (borderline significant, $p = .08$). The authors concluded that there was about 20% difference between acupuncture and placebo. Henry et al. (68), by contrast, demonstrated only a nonsignificant benefit after genuine acupuncture when compared to the mock variety in a trial of 26 migraine patients treated weekly for six weeks. On the other hand, acupuncture seemed more effective than placebo in another randomized crossover trial of 18 Danish patients with refractory chronic tension headaches (69). There was a 31% reduction in pain levels during the active acupuncture.

More recently, another similar trial was reported by Ceccherelli et al. (70), this time of 30 patients with common migraine. Thirteen out of 15 patients given acupuncture and 5 out of 15 patients on placebo treatment were improved. Benefit was sustained for about 20 months in the active patient group and for 3 months in the placebo group.

Despite these modest results, acupuncture may have a role; nevertheless, further trials are needed in less refractory patients, preferably comparing acupuncture with standard drug therapy using a double-placebo design.

MARIJUANA

While the pharmacological properties of cannabis and related substances are now being evaluated and some purified constituents may establish roles in orthodox therapeutics, there has been little systematic work on migraine (71). El Mallakh (72) has reported three patients in whom common migrainous headaches appeared shortly after the abrupt discontinuation of long-term marijuana use. He speculates that this relates to the reported peripheral vasoconstriction and antiplatelet effects of cannabinoids. Whether such substances will ever establish a role in clinical medicine remains to be seen.

SURGICAL TREATMENT

Procedures such as cervical thoracic sympathectomy (73) or trigeminal tractotomy (74) enjoyed popularity before the introduction of any effective drug treatment for migraine, but are no longer considered appropriate. More recently, Koch-Henrichson et al. (75) identified 79 patients suffering from both ill-defined chronic headache and deformity of the nasal septum. They underwent either nasal-reconstructive surgery or observation without treatment. Twenty-seven out of 39 operated patients, but only 7 out of 40 controls, were at least considerably improved after one year, when the authors felt that any placebo effect was likely to have subsided. Unfortunately, the allocation of patients may have been biased, and the trial was not blind. Surgery may be justified for local obstructive symptoms when present, but it can hardly be recommended for the majority of patients with headache rather than local facial pain (76).

More recently, therapeutic embolization of the external carotid circulation was reported in three patients (77). One remained almost symptom-free during one-year follow-up, while another developed headache on the opposite side.

REFERENCES

1. Johnson, E. S. (1983). Patients who chew chrysanthemum leaves, *MIMS Magazine* 15 May: 32-35.
2. Groenwegen, W. A. and Heptinstall, S. (1986). Amounts of feverfew in commercial preparations of the herb. *Lancet, 1*: 44-45.
3. Berry, M. I. (1984). Feverfew faces the future, *Pharmaceutical Journal, 232*: 611-614.
4. Johnson, E. S., Kadam, N. P., Hylands, D. M., and Hylands, P. J. (1985). Efficacy of feverfew as prophylactic treatment of migraine, *Brit. Med. J. 291*: 569-573.
5. Hylands, D. M., Hylands, P. J., Johnson, E. S., Kadam, N. P., and MacRae, K. D. (1985). Efficacy of feverfew as prophylactic treatment of migraine, *Brit. Med. J., 291*: 1128.
6. Kudrow, Personal communication. 1987.

7. Murphy, J. J., Heptinstall, S., and Mitchell, J. R. A. (1988). Randomised double-blind placebo-controlled trial of feverfew in migraine prevention, *Lancet, 2*: 189-192.
8. Lee, K. H., Huang, E. S., Piantadosi, C., Pagano, J. S., and Geissman, T. A. (1971). Cytotoxicity of sesquiterpene lactones, *Cancer Research, 31*: 1649-1654.
9. Collier, H. O. J., Butt, N. M., McDonald-Gibson, W. J., and Saeed, S. A. (1980). Extract of feverfew inhibits prostaglandin biosynthesis, *Lancet, 2*: 922-923.
10. Makheja, A. N. and Bailey, J. M. (1981). The active principle in feverfew, *Lancet, 2*: 1054.
11. Makheja, A. N. and Bailey J. M. (1982). A platelet phospholipase inhibitor from the medical herb feverfew (Tanacetum parthenium), *Prostaglandins, Leukotrienes and Medicine, 8*: 653-660.
12. Heptinstall, S., White, A., Williamson, L., and Mitchell, J. R. A. (1985). Extracts of feverfew inhibit granule secretion in blood platelets and polymorphonuclear leucocytes, *Lancet, 1*: 1071-1074.
13. Groenwegen, W. A., Knight, D. W., and Heptinstall, S. (1986). Compounds extracted from feverfew that have antisecretory activity contain an α-methylene butyrolactone unit, *J. Pharm. Pharmacol., 38*: 709-712.
14. Biggs, M. J., Johnson, E. S., Persaud, N. P., and Ratcliffe, D. M. (1982). Platelet aggregation in patients using feverfew for migraine, *Lancet, 2*: 776.
15. Heptinstall, S., Groenewegen, W. A., Knight, D. W., Spangenberg, P., and Loesche, W. (1987). Studies on feverfew and its mode of action, *Advances in Headache Research* (F.C. Rose, ed.), Libbey, London, pp. 129-134.
16. Hylands, P. J., Hylands, D. M., and Johnson, E. S. (1987). Feverfew in migraine therapy and research, *Migraine: Clinical, Therapeutic, Conceptual and Research Aspects* (J. N. Blau, ed.), Chapman and Hall, London, pp. 543-549.
17. Debney, L. M. and Hedge, A. (1986). Physical trigger factors in migraine—with special reference to weather, *The Prelude to the Migraine Attack* (W. K. Amery and A. Wauquier, eds.), Bailliere Tindall, London, pp. 8-24.
18. Sulman, F. G., Levy, D., Levy, A., Pfeifer, Y., Superstine, E., and Tal, E. (1974). Air-ionometry of hot, dry desert winds (Sharav) and treatment

with air ions of weather-sensitive subjects, *Int. J. Biometeor., 18*: 313-318.
19. Hedge, A. and Eleftharakis, E. (1982). Air ionization: An evaluation of its physiological and psychological effects, *Ann. Occup. Hyg., 25*: 409-419.
20. Hawkins, L. H. (1981). The influence of air ions, temperature and humidity on subjective well-being and comfort, *J. Environmental Psychology, 1*: 279-292.
21. Krueger, A. P. and Reed, E. J. (1976). Biological impact of small air ions, *Science, 193*: 1209-1213.
22. Anthony, M. (1981). "The Effect of Negative Ions on Platelet Serotonin in Normal and Migrainous Subjects," Abstracts of 12th World Congress of Neurology, Kyoto Japan, 1981. Excerpts Medical International Congress, series 548, pp. 84-85.
23. Beardwood, C. J., Abraham, A., and Jordi, P. M. (1986). The effect of exposure to positive space charge on aversive responses to noxious stimuli in rats, *Life Sciences, 39*: 2359-2369.
24. Robertson, A. S., Burge, P. S., Hedge, A., Sims, J., Gills, F. S., Finnegan, M., Pickering, C. A. C., and Dalton, G. (1985). Comparison of health problems related to work and environmental measurements in two office buildings with different ventilation systems, *Brit. Med. J., 291*: 373-376.
25. Finnegan, M. J. and Pickering, C. A. C. (1986). Building-related illness, *Clinical Allergy, 16*: 389-405.
26. Finnegan, M. J., Pickering, C. A. C., Gill, F. S., Ashton, I., and Froese, D. (1987). Effect of negative ion generators in a sick building, *Brit. Med. J., 294*: 1195-1196.
27. Anonymous (1987) Airs, waters, places, *Lancet, 2*: 1062-1063.
28. Peatfield, R. C., Glover, V., Littlewood, J. T., Sandler, M., and Rose, F. C. (1984). The prevalence of diet-induced migraine, *Cephalalgia, 4*: 179-183.
29. Peatfield, R. C. (1989). Pathophysiology and precipitants of migraine, *Migraine in Childhood* (J. M. Hockaday, ed.), Butterworths, London pp. 105-121.
30. Kohlenberg, R. J. (1982). Tyramine sensitivity in dietary migraine: A critical review, *Headache, 22*: 30-34.
31. Hanington, E. (1983). Migraine, *Clinical Reactions to Food* (M. H. Lessof, ed.) Wiley, London, pp. 155-180.

32. Royal College of Physicians (1984). Food intolerance and food aversion, *J. Royal College of Physicians of London, 18*: 83-123.
33. Peatfield, R. C. (1986). Headache, *Clinical Medicine and the Nervous System*, Springer-Verlag, Berlin.
34. Glover, V., Peatfield, R. C., Zammit-Pace, R., Littlewood, J., Gawel, M., Rose, F. C., and Sandler, M. (1981). Platelet monoamine oxidase activity and headache, *J. Neurol. Neurosurg. Psychiatry, 44*: 786-790.
35. Littlewood, J., Glover, V., Sandler, M., Petty, R., Peatfield, R. C., and Rose, F. C. (1982). Platelet phenosulphotransferase deficiency in dietary migraine, *Lancet, 1*: 983-986.
36. Soliman, H., Pradalier, A., Launay, J. M., Dry, J., and Dreux, C. (1987). Decreased phenol and tyramine sulphoconjugation by platelets in dietary migraine. *Advances in Headache Research* (F. C. Rose, ed.), Libbey, London pp. 117-121.
37. Littlewood, J., Gibb, C., Glover, V., Sandler, M., Davies, P. T. G., and Rose, F. C. (1988). Red wine as a cause of migraine, *Lancet, 1*: 558-559.
38. Grant, E. C. G. (1979). Food allergies and migraine, *Lancet, 1*: 966-969.
39. Monro, J., Brostoff, J., Carini, C., and Zilkha, K. (1980). Food allergy in migraine, *Lancet, 2*: 1-4.
40. Egger, J., Carter, C. M., Wilson, J., Turner, M. W., and Soothill, J. F. (1983). Is migraine food allergy? *Lancet, 2*: 865-869.
41. Leviton, A., Slack, W. V., Masek, B., Bana, D., and Graham, J. R. (1984). A computerized behavioral assessment for children with headaches, *Headache, 24*: 182-185.
42. Burn, W. K., Machin, D., and Waters, W. E. (1984). Prevalence of migraine in patients with diabetes, *Brit. Med. J., 289*: 1579-1580.
43. Blau, J. N.. and Pyke, D. A. (1970). Effect of diabetes on migraine, *Lancet, 2*: 241-243.
44. Pearce, J. (1971). Insulin-induced hypoglycemia in migraine, *J. Neurol. Neurosurg. Psychiatry, 34*: 154-156.
45. Hockaday, J. M. (1975). Anomalies of carbohydrate metabolism, *Modern Topics in Migraine* (J. Pearce, ed.), Heinemann, London, pp. 124-137.
46. Hunter, C. R. and Mayfield, F. H. (1949). Role of the upper cervical roots in the production of pain in the head. *Am. J. Surg., 78*: 743-749.

47. Kerr, F. W. L. (1961). Structural relation of the trigeminal spinal tract upper cervical roots and the solitary nucleus in the cat, *Experimental Neurology, 4*: 134-148.
48. Edmeads, J. (1978). Headaches and head pains associated with diseases of the cervical spine, *Medical Clinics of North America, 62*: 533-544.
49. Bogduk, N., Corrigan, B., Kelly, P., Schneider, G., and Farr, R. (1985). Cervical headache, *Med. J. of Australia, 143*: 202-207.
50. Pfaffenrath, V., Dandekar, R., and Pollmann, W. (1987). Cervicogenic headache—the clinical picture, radiological findings and hypotheses on its pathophysiology, *Headache, 27*: 495-499.
51. Bogduk,N. and Marsland, A. (1986). On the concept of third occipital headache, *J. Neurol. Neurosurg. Psychiatry, 49*: 775-780.
52. Ehni, G. and Benner, B. Occipital neuralgia and the C1-2 arthrosis syndrome, *J. Neurosurg, 61*: 961-965.
53. Bogduk, N. (1981). Local anesthetic blocks of the second cervical ganglion: A technique with application in occipital headache, *Cephalalgia, 1*: 41-50.
54. Bogduk, N. (1985). The anatomy of occipital neuralgia, *Clinical and Experimental Neurology, 21*: 167-184.
55. Mealy, K., Brennan, H., and Fenelon, G. C. C. Early mobilization of acute whiplash injuries, *Brit. Med. J., 292*: 656-657.
56. Anthony, M. (1987). The role of the occipital nerve in unilateral headache, *Advances in Headache Research* (F. C. Rose, ed.), Libbey, London, pp. 257-262.
57. Parker, G. B., Tupling, H., and Pryor, D. S. (1978). A controlled trial of cervical manipulation for migraine, *Aust.-NZ J. Med., 8*: 589-593.
58. Costen, J. B. (1936). Neuralgias and ear symptoms, *JAMA, 107*: 252-255.
59. Thomson, H. (1971). Mandibular dysfunction syndrome, *Brit. Dent. J., 130*:187-193.
60. Feinmann, C., Harris, M., and Cawley, R. (1984). Psychogenic facial pain: Presentation and treatment, *Brit. Med. J., 288*: 436-438.
61. Leviton, A. and Camenga, D. (1969). Migraine associated with hyper-pre-beta lipoproteinemia, *Neurology, 19*: 963-966.
62. Glueck, C. J. and Bates, S. R. (1986). Migraine in children: Association with primary and familial dyslipoproteinemias, *Pediatrics, 77*: 316-321.

63. Glueck, C. J., McCarren, T., Hitzemann, R., Allen, C., Hogg, E., Kloss, R., Thompson, B., Yunker, R., Gartside, P., and Lazkarzewski, P. M. (1986). Amelioration of severe migraine with omega-3 fatty acids: A double-blind, placebo-controlled clinical trial. *Amer. J. Clinical Nutrition, 43*: 710A.
64. Marwick, C. (1987). Article brings censure recommendation, *JAMA, 258*: 1137.
65. Anonymous (1988). Fish Oil, *Lancet, 1*: 1081-1083.
66. Loh, L., Nathan, P. W., Schott, G. D., and Zilkha, K. J. Acupuncture versus medical treatment for migraine and muscle tension headaches, *J. Neurol. Neurosurg. Psychiatry, 47*: 333-337.
67. Dowson, D. I., Lewith, G. T., and Machin, D. (1985). The effects of acupuncture versus placebo in the treatment of headache, *Pain, 21*: 35-42.
68. Henry, P., Baille, H. M., Dartigues, J. F., and Jogeix, M. (1985). Headaches and acupuncture, *Updating in Headache* (V. Pfaffenrath, P. O. Lundberg, and O. Sjaastad, eds.), Springer-Verlag, Berlin, pp. 208-216.
69. Hansen, P. E. and Hansen, J. H. (1985). Acupuncture treatment of chronic tension headache—a controlled crossover trial, *Cephalalgia, 5*: 137-142.
70. Cecceriell, F., Ambrosio, F., Avila, M., Duse, G., Munari, A., and Giron, G. P. Acupuncture vs. placebo in the common migraine: A double-blind study, *Cephalalgia, 7(Suppl. 6)*: 499-500.
71. Hollister, L. E. (1986). Health aspects of cannabis, *Pharmacological Reviews, 38*: 1-20.
72. El-Mallakh, R. S. (1987). Marijuana and migraine, *Headache, 27*: 442-443.
73. Love, J. G. and Adson, A. W. (1936). Effect of cervicothoracic sympathectomy on headaches, *Arch. Neurol., 35*: 1203-1207.
74. Olivecrona, H. (1947) Notes on the surgical treatment of migraine, *Acta Medica Scand., Suppl. 196*: 229-237.
75. Koch-Henriksen, N., Gammelgaard, N., Hvidegaard, T., and Stoksted, P. (1984) Chronic headache: The role of deformity of the nasal septum, *Brit. Med. J., 288*: 434-435.
76. Pearce, J. (1984). Chronic headache: The role of deformity of the nasal septum, *Brit. Med. J., 288*: 1005.
77. Horton, J. and Kerber, C. W. (1985). Therapeutic embolization for vascular headache, *Amer. J. Neuroradiology, 6*: 299.

Index

Abdominal migraine, 168
Abortive treatment, 45-55
  analgesics, 51-52
  aura without headache (migraine equivalents), 53-54
  corticosteroids, 52-53
  ergotamine-rebound headache, 50-51
  nonpharmacologic therapy, 46
  sedatives and antiemetics, 52
  status migrainosus, 53
  vasoconstrictive agents, 46-50
Acupuncture, 250-251
Acute confusional migraine in children, 201-202
Air ionization, 243-244
Alcohol, 7, 32, 35
Alice in Wonderland syndrome, 198
Alternating hemiplegia, 203
Altitude changes, 40-41, 43
Amitriptyline, 206, 207-208
  versus propranolol (comparative study), 77-78

Analgesics, 51-52
Anticonvulsants, 208
Antiemetics, 48, 52
Anti-inflammatory agents, 48
  See also Nonsteroidal anti-inflammatory agents (NSAIDs)
Antimigraine medications in the elderly, contraindications to, 184
Antiplatelet aggregating agents, 134-137
  aspirin, 135-136
  dazoxiben, 136-137
  dipyridamole, 137
  sulfinpyrazone, 136
Artificial sweeteners, 37
Aspartame, 37
Aspirin, 135-136, 138
  versus propranolol (comparative study), 76-77
Atenolol, 75
Atherothrombotic vascular disease as cause of headache in the elderly, 178-181

260 Index

Aura:
 depression and, 15-16
 migraine with, 4-6, 191
 migraine without, 3-4, 53-54, 191
 prolonged, migraine with, 158
 sequence of headache and, 17-18
Autogenic feedback, 214-215
Autonomic dysfunctions accompanying migraine, 168
 effect of beta blockers on, 61-62

Baked goods, 33
Basilar migraine (BM), 5-6, 159-161
 in children, 201
Beta blockers, 22, 57-86
 autonomic dysregulation, 61-62
 beta subtype selectivity, 58-59
 central catecholamine actions, 62-63
 cerebral circulation, 60-61
 central nervous system penetration, 60
 membrane-stabilizing activity, 60
 partial agonist activity, 59
 pharmacology, 57-58, 65-81
  beta-adrenergic-blocking agents with partial agonist activity, 75-81
  case reports and open studies, 66-69
  controlled trials comparing beta blockers with propranolol, 81
  double-blind placebo-controlled studies, 69-75
  studies of beta-adrenergic-blocking agents, 65-66
 plasma levels, 64-65

[Beta blockers]
 platelet studies, 63-64
 serotonin antagonistic effects, 59-60
Beverages, 33
Biochemical concepts of migraine, 19-22
 catecholamines and serotonin, 19-22
 other biochemicals, 21-22
 substance P, 20-21
Biofeedback therapy, 213-238
 considerations in selecting biofeedback therapists, 230-232
 considerations in selecting patients for treatment, 224-230
  age, 224-225
  cost, 229-230
  finding time, 225-226
  frequency and number of sessions, 226
  less responsive types, 227-228
  nonspecific benefits, 228-229
  personality factors, 226-227
  side effects, 228
 in the larger treatment context, 232-233
 mechanisms of, 222-224
 in relation to medical therapy, 219-222
Blood flow regulation, 14
Blood-volume pulse (BVP) feedback, 215-216
Building sickness, 244-245

Caffeine, 8, 32, 35-36
 sources of, 37
Calcium channel blockers (CCBs), 22, 99-125, 208

Index

[Calcium channel blockers (CCBs)]
  comparison of, 115-118
    efficacy, 118
    side effects, 119
  pharmacology of, 101-115
    diltiazem, 108
    flunarizine, 113-114
    nifedipine, 108-109
    nimodipine, 108-112
    verapamil, 101-108
  role of calcium in vascular smooth muscle, 99-101
Captopril, 147
Carbamazepine, 78
Catecholamines, 19-20
  beta blockers actions on, 62-63
Central nervous system (CNS), beta blockers ability to prenetrate, 60
Cerebral circulation, effect of beta blockers on, 60-61
Cerebrovascular tone, regulation of, 14
Cervical spondylosis as cause of headache in the elderly, 176
Children, 189-212
  biofeedback therapy and, 224-225
  classification and etiology, 191
  epidemiology, 190-191
  evaluation, 191-194
  headache data base, 192
  history, 189-190
  migraine substrate and, 196-198
  migraine syndrome and, 195-196
  migraine variants and, 202-204
  pathophysiology, 194-195
  prognosis, 208-209
  treatment, 204-208
  types of migraine, 202-208

Chocolate, 7, 33
Classic migraine (migraine with aura), 4-6, 191
  in children, 197-198
  IHS diagnostic criteria for, 11-12
Clonidine, 78, 146-147
  beta blockers versus (comparative study), 78-79
Cluster headache, 1
Cold packs, 46
Common migraine (migraine without aura), 3-4, 53-54, 191
  in children, 197-198, 199
  IHS diagnostic criteria for, 9-10
Complicated migraine, 6, 157-158, 191
  in children, 200
  treatment of, 166-167
  See also types of complicated migraine
Corticosteroids, 52-53
Cyclandelate, 147
Cyproheptadine, 59, 133, 206-207

Dairy products, 33
Dazoxiben, 136-137
Depression, 42
  aura of classic migraine and, 15-16
Desserts, 33
Diagnosis of migraine, 2-12
  diagnostic criteria, 9-12
  family, social, and psychological history, 9
  history of prior treatment, 8-9
  migraine with aura (classic migraine), 4-6
  migraine without aura (common migraine), 3-4

[Diagnosis of migraine]
  patient history, 2
  provocative factors, 7-8
Diet, 31-38, 245-246
  alcohol, 35
  caffeine, 35-36
  fasting, 36
  monosodium glutamate (MSG), 34
  other foods, 37-38
  phenylethylamine, 35
  sodium nitrite, 34
  tyramine, 32-34
Dihydroergotamine mesylate, 146-147
Diltiazem, 108
  efficacy of, 118
  side effects of, 119
Dipyridamole, 137
Dopaminergic agonists, 145

Elderly, the, 173-188
  biofeedback therapy for, 224-225
  lesions producing headache in, 177
  problems of treatment for, 183-185
  size of migraine problem for, 174-183
Electrical stimulation, 46
Environmental sources, 40-41, 43
Epilepsy-equivalent syndrome, 204
Ergot alkaloids,
  dihydroergotamine mesylate, 144-145
  ergotamine tartrate, 141-143
Ergotamine-rebound headache, 50-51

Ergotamine tartrate, 46, 48, 141-143
Estrogen replacement, 40
Exertion, 42

(Familial) hemiplegic migraine, 5, 158-159
Fasting, 36
Femoxitine, 133-134
Fenoprofen, 139-140
Feverfew, 239-243
Fish, 33
Flunarizine, 113-114
  efficacy of, 118
  side effects of, 119
Food:
  migraine-precipitating, 7-8, 33, 245-246
  See also Diet
Fruits, 33

Giant-cell arteritis and cause of headache in the elderly, 178

Hand-warming biofeedback, 215, 216
Headache-related distress, 227
Hemiplegia, alternating, 11
Hemiplegic migraine, 5, 158-159
  in children, 200
Hormonal influences on migraine, 38-40
  estrogen replacement, 40
  oral contraceptives, 39
  pregnancy, 39-40

Index

5-Hydroxyindoleacectic acid (5-HIAA), 19
Hypoglycemia, 246-247

Increased intracranial pressure (IICP), 193
Indomethacin, 138-139
Initiation of a migraine attack, 22-23
International Headache Society:
  diagnostic criteria for migraine with aura, 11-12
  diagnostic criteria for migraine without aura, 9-10
Interval therapy, 148-149
Intrinsic sympathomimetic activity, 58
Isometheptene mucate, 48, 49-50

Ketoprofen, 139-140

Marijuana, 251
Meat, 7, 33
Medications:
  antimigraine, contraindications to (for the elderly), 184
  biofeedback therapy combined with, 219-222
  that provoke migraine, 8
  in the elderly, 181, 182
Mefenamic acid, 140-141
Membraine-stabilizing activity of beta blockers, 60
Menstrual migraine, 7
Meta-analysis of biofeedback and relaxation therapy, 217-219
Methysergide, 59, 229-232

Metoprolol
  double-blind placebo-controlled study, 74-75
  pizotifen versus (comparative study), 77
Migraine equivalents, 6, 53-54, 167-168
  treatment of, 169
Migraine sine-hemicrania, 203-204
Migraine variants, 191
  in children, 202-204
Migraine with aura (classic migraine), 4-6, 191
  in children, 197-198
  IHS diagnostic criteria for, 11-12
Migraine without aura (common migraine), 3-4, 53-54,
  in children, 197-198, 199
  IHS diagnostic criteria for, 9-10
Migraine with prolonged aura (MPA), 158
Migrainous infarction, 163-166
Monosodium glutamate (MSG), 7, 32, 34
Muscular contraction, headache due to, 1

Nadolol:
  case study, 68-69
  double-blind placebo-controlled study, 72-73
Naproxen, 139-140
Naproxen sodium, 139-140
Neck structure, treatment of, 247-249
Neural theories of migraine, 14-19
  aura and spreading depression, 15-16

[Neural theories of migraine]
  headache and the trigeminal nerve, 16-17
  sequence of aura and headache, 17-18
  triggering pathways, 18-19
Nifedipine, 108-109
  efficacy of, 118
  side effects of, 110
Nimodipine, 97-100, 109-112
  efficacy of, 106, 118
  side effects of, 112, 119
Nonpharmacologic therapy, 46
Nonsteroidal anti-inflammatory agents (NSAIDs), 48, 51, 137-141, 208
  aspirin, 138
  fenoprofen, 139-140
  indomethacin, 138-139
  ketoprofen, 139-140
  mefenamic acid, 140-141
  naproxen, 139-140
  naproxen sodium, 139-140
  propranolol versus (comparative study), 80-81
  tolfenamic acid, 140-141

Ophthalmoplegic migraine, 5, 161-162
  in children, 200-201
Oral contraceptives, 39

Parenteral therapy for status migrainosus, 53
Paroxysmal torticollis, 202
Paroxysmal vertigo, 202
Pathophysiologic headaches, two types of, 1-2

Pathophysiology of migraine, 12-24
  biochemical concepts of migraine, 19-22
  initiation of a migraine attack, 22-23
  mechanisms of other features of a migraine, 23-24
  neural theories, 14-19
  platelets and migraine, 13-14
  regulation of cerebrovascular tone and blood flow, 14
  relevance to therapy, 22
  summary of neurovascular biochemical changes, 24
  vascular theories, 12-13
Phenylethylamine, 7, 35
Pindolol, 78
Pizotifen, 132
  metoprolol versus (comparative study), 77
Plasma lipids, manipulation of, 249-250
Platelet dysfunction, 13-14
  effect of beta blockers on, 63-64
Positron emission tomography (PET), 16
Precipitating causes of migraine, 31-44
  altitude changes, 40-41, 43
  diet, 31-38
    alcohol, 35
    caffeine, 35-36
    fasting, 36
    monosodium glutamate (MSG), 34
    other foods, 37-38
    phenylethylamine, 35
    sodium nitrite, 34
    tyramine, 32-34

Index

[Precipitating causes of migraine]
  environmental factors, 43
  exertion, 42
  hormonal influences, 38-40
    estrogen replacement, 40
    oral contraceptives, 39
    pregnancy, 39-40
  psychologic factors, 41-42
  weather, 40, 43
Pregnancy, 39-40
Processed meats, 7
Propranolol, 206, 207
  amitriptyline versus (comparative study), 77-78
  aspirin versus (comparative study), 76-77
  case study of, 66-68
  controlled trials comparing beta blockers with, 81
  double-blind placebo-controlled study, 69-72
  NSAIDs versus, 80-81
Prostaglandin inhibitors, 22
Psychic migraine, 168

Rebound headache due to ergotamine treatment, 50-51
Respiratory disease as cause of headache in the elderly, 181-183
Retinal migraine, 5, 163, 168

Sedatives, 52
Serotonin, 19-20
Serotonin antagonists, 59-60, 128-134
  beta blockers versus (comparative study), 79-80

[Serotonin antagonists]
  cyproheptadine, 133
  femoxitine, 133-134
  methysergide, 129-132
  pizotifen, 132
Serotonin precursors, 145
Side effects:
  of biofeedback therapy, 228
  of calcium channel blockers, 107, 112, 119
Sodium nitrite, 32, 34
Status migrainosus, 53
Steroids, 48
Stress, 42
Substance P, 20-21
Sulfinpyrazine, 136
Suloctidil, 146
Surgical treatment, 252

Temporomandibular joint disease, 249
Tension headaches, 1
Timolol:
  case study of, 68
  double-blind placebo-controlled study, 73-74
Tolfenamic acid, 140-141
Transient migrainous accompaniments (TMAs), 163-167
  in the elderly, 175-176
Trigeminal nerve, 16-17
Triggering pathways, 18-19, 196-198
Tyramine, 32-34

Unproven therapeutic measures, 239-257
  acupuncture, 250-251

[Unproven therapeutic measures]
  air ionization, 243-244
  building sickness and, 244-245
  feverfew, 239-243
  food allergy and, 245-246
  hypoglycemia and, 246-247
  manipulation of plasma lipids, 249-250
  marijuana, 251
  surgical treatment, 252
  temporomandibular joint disease and, 249
  treatment of neck structures, 247-249

Vanillymandelic acid (VMA), 20
Vascular hypertension as cause of headache in the elderly, 176-178
Vascular theories of migraine, 12-13
Vasoconstrictive agents, 46-50
Vegetables, 33
Verapamil, 101-108
  clinical studies with, 104-108
  efficacy of, 118
  pharmacology of, 101-104
  side effects of, 107, 119

Weather, 40, 43

About the Editor

SEYMOUR DIAMOND is Director of the Diamond Headache Clinic and of the Inpatient Headache Unit, Louis A. Weiss Medical Hospital, Chicago, Illinois, and Adjunct Professor of Pharmacology and Molecular Biology at the Chicago Medical School, North Chicago, Illinois. The author or coauthor of over 260 journal articles and over 20 books, he is a member of numerous professional organizations including the International Association for the study of Pain, International Headache Society, American Academy of Pain Medicine, American Association for the Study of Headache, American Society for Clinical Therapeutics and Pharmacology, and American Medical Association. He is Executive Officer, Research Group on Migraine and Headache, World Federation of Neurology, and Executive Director, National Headache Foundation. Dr. Diamond received the M.B. (1948) and M.D. (1949) degrees from the Chicago Medical School, Illinois.